# *Book of Dreams*

*Oneiromancy and Medical Astrology*

SKY MEDICINE SERIES

*Book of Dreams*

*is Volume IX in the Sky Medicine series*

SKY MEDICINE

# *Book of Dreams*

## *Oneiromancy and Medical Astrology*

William Morris, DAOM, PhD

ISBN: 978-1-942694-01-4 (hardcover)
ISBN: 978-1-942694-02-1 (paperback)
ISBN: 978-1-942694-03-8 (ebook)

First Edition

Typeset in Palatino Linotype

33 Publishing
Austin, TX 78701

While modern technology assisted in the structural synthesis of the historical data within these pages, the medical insights and esoteric interpretations remain an original work of clinical alchemy. This volume represents the author's lifelong dedication to the marriage of tradition and creative scholarship.

**Medical and Professional Disclaimer** This book is intended for informational and educational purposes only and does not constitute medical advice, diagnosis, or treatment. Although the author is a licensed healthcare provider, the historical, astrological, and herbal material presented herein is for scholarly exploration and does not establish a provider-patient relationship.

By using this book, the reader acknowledges that they possess the appropriate professional training, licensure, and clinical judgment necessary to evaluate and apply any information within their legal scope of practice. The historical and traditional protocols discussed must be cross-referenced with modern safety standards and clinical guidelines. Readers who are not licensed healthcare providers should consult a qualified professional before implementing any changes.

The author and 33 Publishing disclaim all liability for any loss, injury, or risk, personal or otherwise, incurred as a consequence, directly or indirectly, of the use and application of any of the contents of this book.

*For Theresa*
*who walks with me between the worlds*

*τὰ μεγάλα πάντα διὰ ὀνειράτων καὶ μαντείας θεοῖς προσήκει*
*"All great things are revealed to humanity through dreams and prophecy."*

—Plato, *Phaedrus* 244a

To the lineage of the healers and the wisdom of the stars: This volume is offered as an act of creative scholarship and deep clinical devotion. Protected by forty-five years of clinical attention and the direct mentorship of the masters, these pages carry the 'Shakti' of a living tradition. May this work remain an inviolable bridge between the ancient and the emergent, serving the soul of the practitioner and the life of the patient.

# Contents

## APPENDICES

# List of Tables

# Preface

Every night, the gates open. The conscious mind releases its grip; the soul slips its moorings and travels. What it encounters there—the images, warnings, visitations—has occupied humanity's attention since we first gathered around fires to share what the night had shown us.

Oneiromancy—from Greek ὄνειρος (dream) and μαντεία (divination)—names the ancient art of reading destiny in the theater of sleep. The practice treats the sleeping mind as oracle, the dream as letter from the unseen world. Where the soul travels unmoored from waking constraint, it speaks in symbol and portent; oneiromancy is the discipline of listening.

The present volume emerges following forty-five years of clinical practice at the intersections of astrology, Classical Chinese Medicine, and homeopathy. Traditional astrological methods for assessing dream significance, Chinese medical frameworks that read dream content as the voice of the organ-spirits, the Vedic understanding of karmic residue surfacing in sleep, the deep history of incubation temples where pilgrims sought healing through divinely sent visions—each tradition takes dreams seriously, distinguishes vision from noise, connects individual experience to heavenly realms.

The Western astrological tradition, transmitted through the medieval Arabic synthesis and codified by Guido Bonatti, developed protocols for determining whether a dream conveyed true prophecy or phantasm. These methods center on the ninth house—the *Domus Dei*—employing essential dignities, planetary conditions, and aspectual relationships to assess veracity. Classical Chinese Medicine approaches dreams differently: the five-spirit framework locates psychic functions in specific organ systems, with the *hún* of the Liver bearing particular responsibility for dream activity.

The dream becomes data—not prediction but expression, the organ-spirits speaking in the only language available to them. The

Vedic tradition locates dream signification in the twelfth house while examining the ninth for prophetic capacity. Here the dream opens onto karma itself, revealing what approaches and what might yet be averted.

Sky Medicine synthesizes these traditions without collapsing their differences. The work is transdisciplinary—tracing dream practice across cultures and periods, developing awareness of omenology and spiritual transformation, illuminating conditions of life as dreams reveal them. The dream time offers tools of transformation and healing; the book explores them.

Fourteen chapters trace oneiromancy through its major transmissions: Mesopotamian court interpreters, Aboriginal Dreamtime, the shaking medicine of the Kalahari, Indigenous vision quests, Egyptian threshold consciousness, Vedic frameworks of validation and timing, Classical Chinese Medicine's organ-spirit diagnostics and Daoist sleep cultivation, Bön dream yoga as bardo preparation, the Greek synthesis from Artemidorus through the Asclepian temples, the Persian-Arabic transmission culminating in Bonatti's veracity protocols, syncretic integration, and ethnobotanical allies. Appendices provide reference tables, therapeutic protocols, and mantric formulas.

The dream remains what the ancients knew it to be—a letter from the depths, a communication from powers that speak when the daylight mind falls silent. Such letters require reading. The skills can be taught. The failure to attend carries consequences.

The gates open nightly. Enter prepared.

William Morris
Kootenay Lake, British Columbia Winter Solstice, 2025

# Note on Method and Scope

Sky Medicine works across traditions. The sources assembled here—Hellenistic, Vedic, Classical Chinese, Hermetic, Paracelsian—are living technologies refined across millennia by practitioners facing the same clinical realities we face. Fidelity to these traditions means engaging their generative problems, not merely their received solutions.

The method is transdisciplinary. Different civilizations observed the same sky and the same human body. When Greek medical astrology, Vedic timing techniques, and Chinese circulatory theory produce overlapping protocols, we confront convergent discovery rather than coincidence. Their parallel findings carry weight.

Clinical outcomes remain the final arbiter. Forty-five years of practice inform every synthesis here. Where traditions conflict, the consulting room adjudicates. Where they converge, confidence increases. Where gaps appear, original formulations emerge—extensions of living inquiry rather than departures from tradition.

The frameworks presented reflect the author's direct training and initiatory transmission in Classical Chinese Medicine, Vedic and Western astrology, Āyurveda, and herbal medicine. Traditions beyond this scope appear as fellow travelers in celestial medicine, awaiting practitioners who will extend the synthesis further, and as an invitation to practice.

# Acknowledgments

No work emerges in isolation. What is systematized here flows through lineages older than any of us, transmitted by practitioners who understood that what they carried was not theirs to keep but theirs to pass on.

My training in Traditional Chinese Medicine at Emperor's College provided the theoretical foundation for understanding dreams as expressions of the organ-spirits. The California Institute of Integral Studies, where I completed my doctorate in Transformative Studies, offered the transdisciplinary framework that makes synthesis across medical, astrological, and contemplative traditions methodologically rigorous rather than merely eclectic.

Certain teachers shaped this work through direct transmission.

John H.F. Shen and Leon Hammer transmitted the Menghe-Ding pulse lineage that informs the clinical chapters of this volume. At Dr. Shen's passing in 2000, I received what I can only describe as a spiritual transmission—an electrical sensation throughout the body, an overwhelming sense of his presence, a direct communication in which he offered the spiritual power of the teachings he had carried. He connected me to what the Menghe tradition calls the "blood river of teaching." That transmission continues. My 1986 study with Professor Ding Jie Ming opened a parallel channel into the same tradition.

Ron Teeguarden transmitted the Daoist tonic tradition of Grandmaster Sung Jin Park, Keeper of Rites of Kook Sun Do.

Lee Lehman's pioneering excavation of traditional astrological medicine opened pathways I continue to walk after twelve years of study.

Bradford Keeney, my dissertation chair, initiated me into the shaking medicine of the Kalahari San—a lineage that fundamentally shaped my understanding of dreams as communal healing phenomena.

My Jyotiṣa guru, Pt. Sanjay Rath, teaches the Vedic tradition through the Śrī Jagannāth Center; his publicly available teachings inform Part Four.

Maa Gyaan Suveera transmits the lineage of Swami Samarth, whose teachings on sādhanā and divine grace inform the contemplative dimensions of this work.

Beyond these named teachers, I have received initiations across Egyptian, Hermetic, alchemical, Pythagorean, Daoist, Śaiva, Reiki, Advaitin, Vaiṣṇava, Buddhist, Kabbalistic, and Western Mystery traditions. These confer no degrees, satisfy no licensing requirements. They are acknowledged because they shape how this material is understood and transmitted.

Theresa Lee has supported this work in ways too numerous to catalog. The dedication does not adequately address that debt.

AI language models assisted with research organization and editorial synthesis; all intellectual content, protocols, and interpretations are solely the author's work.

The lineages named here do not exhaust the transmissions that shaped this work. Whatever merit this volume possesses belongs to those who preserved and transmitted what is systematized here. Its errors remain my own.

May this work serve the traditions that made it possible. May it reach those who need it. May the gates continue to open.

# Note on Transliteration and Conventions

This work draws upon ancient lineages, but its aim is the restoration of health and the awakening of vision. Transliteration conventions prioritize clinical resonance over rigid scholarly apparatus. These terms are not artifacts of the past but living keys for the clinic and the soul.

## Chinese Terms

Chinese terms appear in Hànyǔ Pīnyīn with tone diacriticals (ā, á, ǎ, à). Traditional characters accompany terms at first occurrence for readers who want them; they are not essential to following the material. All Chinese terms are italicized.

The five organ-spirits (*wǔ shén* 五神) appear throughout:

*hún* 魂 — ethereal soul (Liver, Wood, Jupiter) *pò* 魄 — corporeal soul (Lung, Metal, Venus) *shén* 神 — spirit-consciousness (Heart, Fire, Mars) *yì* 意 — intellect-intention (Spleen, Earth, Saturn) *zhì* 志 — will-purpose (Kidney, Water, Mercury)

Other recurring terms include *qì* 氣 (vital energy), *yīn* 陰 and *yáng* 陽 (the complementary polarities), and *zàng* 臟 (the five yin organs).

## Sanskrit Terms

Sanskrit terms appear in IAST transliteration with standard diacriticals:

*Jyotiṣa* — Vedic astrology *nakṣatra* — lunar mansion *daśā* — planetary period system *Āruḍha Lagna* — significator of manifest appearance

## General Conventions

The glossary provides consolidated definitions for quick reference.

# How to Use This Book

*The Book of Dreams* draws on multiple traditions—Western astrological, Classical Chinese medical, Vedic. A glossary organized by cultural section appears at the end of the volume. Four pathways open here:

*Western Astrologers*

Chapters Eleven and Twelve (ninth house protocols, Bonatti's veracity rules), then Appendices B–D (dignities, planetary hours, Almuten calculation). This ground prepares the Chinese and Vedic material that follows.

*Chinese Medicine Practitioners*

Part Two (Chapters Six through Eight): the *wǔ shén* framework, five-flavor therapeutics, spirit disturbance patterns, Daoist sleep cultivation. The astrological chapters then reveal how planetary conditions speak through familiar organ-spirit dynamics.

*Vedic Astrologers*

Chapter Five (twelfth house, the four watches, *nakṣatra* timing, karmic interpretation), then Appendices E–F (Ārūḍha Lagna calculation, lunar mansions). The Western chapters present parallel methods—ninth house emphasis alongside twelfth house—that deepen *Jyotiṣa* practice.

*General Readers and Depth Psychologists*

Chapters One and Two (historical foundations, cross-cultural dream practices), then Chapter Thirteen (processing methods including Jungian, Gestalt, and Focusing techniques). Technical chapters await when curiosity calls; the glossary orients unfamiliar terms.

Chapters cross-reference one another and may be read in any order. The threefold method—Western, Chinese, and Vedic working together—weaves throughout. Technical terms receive brief parenthetical definitions at first occurrence; the glossary provides fuller treatment. The Oneirobotany chapter (Fourteen) becomes practical reference once the interpretive ground is laid.

# Part One

# Foundations

*πάντα γὰρ τὰ μεγάλα ἐπισφαλῆ*

**"All great things are perilous."**

—Plato, *Republic* 497d

Before technique, orientation. Before protocol, the recognition that dreams have always mattered—that humanity's oldest records preserve not only what people dreamed but how they distinguished vision from noise, prophecy from digestion, divine message from demonic interference.

The two chapters that follow establish the ground on which all subsequent traditions build. The first surveys the major oneiromantic systems, mapping the spectrum from external (divine communication) to internal (organ-spirit expression) that organizes this volume. The second recovers what literate civilizations inherited from oral cultures: the understanding that dreams belong to communities before they belong to dreamers, and that the night sky governs what sleep delivers.

## Chapter One

# An Historical Overview of Oneiromancy

*ἐκ Διός ἐστιν ὄνειρος*

"The dream is from Zeus."

—Homer, Iliad I.63

## Etymology and Definition

Oneiromancy—from Greek *oneiros* (dream) and *manteia* (divination)—is the art of interpreting dreams for prophetic or diagnostic purposes. The term first appears in Artemidorus of Daldis during the second century CE, though the practice reaches back to the earliest documented civilizations. Every major healing tradition developed methods for interpreting this nightly visitation—recognizing in dreams a form of communication that transcends ordinary sensory experience.

Dream interpretation appears in every documented culture. Whether divine message, ancestral visitation, organ-spirit wandering, or karmic disclosure—dreams present images that demand reading. How to read them, how to ground the interpretation—these questions occupied healers across millennia.

## The Pan-Celestial Framework

The *History and Foundations of Medical Astrology* volume in this series establishes the pan-celestial thesis: celestial medicine represents a universal human response to the observation of cycles. Different cultures accessed the same sky and translated it into culturally specific medical idioms. Multiple traditions developed astronomical observation independently—or from shared heritage so ancient it precedes written record—and applied celestial principles to healing through distinctive physiological frameworks.

The oneiromantic traditions surveyed in this volume demonstrate the pan-celestial principle in a specific domain. Dreams and stars belong together—both are heavenly writing that trained interpreters can read. Yet how each tradition reads that writing—and where it locates the sky's influence—ranges from fully external to fully internal.

### *The External-Internal Spectrum*

Mesopotamian oneiromancy stands at the external pole. Dreams arrive as messages from deities—communications from outside the dreamer, requiring ritual response. The dream-god Zaqīqu blows divine messages into the passive sleeper like wind. Interpretation serves the state; remediation involves protective ritual to redirect fate.

Egyptian oneiromancy stands at the threshold. The dream (*resut*) is an "awakening" into liminal space where external divine communication meets internal constitutional reception. The Horus/Seth typology recognizes that the same message registers differently depending on the dreamer's inherent nature. The Four Sons of Horus map received influence to specific organs. External message meets embodied constitution.

Chinese oneiromancy stands at the internal pole. Dreams arise from the condition of the five organ-spirits (*wǔ shén*). The ethereal soul (*hún*) generates dream experience through its nocturnal wandering. The sky has been fully internalized—the Eight Extraordinary Vessels serve as internal wiring for celestial influences. Dream diagnosis reads the movement of *shén* through the *zàng-fǔ* organ systems. Not omen-reading but diagnosis—the body speaking through dream.

Indian and Greek traditions occupy intermediate positions, each with distinctive features explored in subsequent chapters. The integration presented in later chapters does not homogenize these approaches. It provides a way to navigate parallel systems—each accessing the same sky through its own physiological language.

## Mesopotamian Foundations

The oldest surviving dream interpretation texts come from Mesopotamia, where dreams belonged to the omen system that structured Babylonian and Assyrian thought. Dreams occupied the same category as celestial omens, extispicy (divination by entrails), and other forms of divine communication. The dream-god Zaqīqu—whose name means "to blow"—carried divine messages like wind into the sleeper's mind. The same gods who arranged the stars and marked the sacrificial liver also sent dreams. Dreams and stars belonged together: both were *šiṭir šamê*, heavenly writing that trained interpreters could read.

### *The Iškar Zaqīqu: Structure and Method*

The *Iškar Zaqīqu*, the Series of the Dream-God, comprises eleven tablets compiled during the seventh century BCE from older sources. The central tablets (II–IX) use protasis-apodosis format—"If a man dreams X, then Y will occur"—the same conditional logic governing all Mesopotamian omen literature. The framing tablets (I, X, XI) preserve ritual procedures—the therapeutic dimension.

The Assyrian dream-masters understood that the gods were master poets, weaving destiny through wordplay. When a dreamer encountered *miḫru*-wood, the Divine Scribe was punning on the dreamer's future, ensuring they would stand without rival. These were not coincidences of sound but intentional signatures placed within the soul's sleep to signal shifting fortune. To interpret a dream was to read the puns of the gods.

Mesopotamian divination distinguished between solicited omens (provoked by ritual) and unsolicited omens (spontaneous signs, including dreams). This empirical approach established a precedent that echoes through every tradition since. The modern astrologer consulting traditional texts for planetary significations participates in the same mode of knowing.

## *The Exorcist-Priest and Apotropaic Ritual*

When a dream portended ill, the priest-exorcist (*āšipu*) performed protective rituals preserved in Tablets I, X, and XI. These procedures dissolved the connection between omen and outcome: transferring the portent to effigy or substitute object, ritual bathing to wash away pollution, aromatic fumigation to drive away malevolent *zaqīqu* spirits.

The *namburbi* (releasing) rituals dissolved the omen's power. The dream's warning was a prognosis, not a fate; an appropriate ritual response could redirect what was to come. Ritual remediation persists in later traditions—threatening dreams addressed through talisman, herb, or devotion. Diagnosis implies prognosis; prognosis enables intervention.

## *Gula and the Somatic Dimension*

The goddess Gula governed healing and biliary function—the condition of the bile thought to regulate dream quality. A disturbed liver produced disturbed dreams; a settled digestive system permitted clear reception. Here the external model bends inward: the body's condition affects receptivity to divine message, even when the message originates outside.

Gula's celestial home was the constellation The Goat (MUL $UZ_3$), corresponding to modern Lyra with its brilliant star Vega. Her sacred dog occupied the neighboring constellation MUL $UR.GI_7$ in what we now call Hercules—healer and companion paired in the summer sky. Temple practices at Gula's sanctuaries included placing patients under the stars overnight to receive her healing influence, a form of celestial incubation that preceded later traditions.

## Egyptian Oneiromancy

The Egyptian understanding of dream experience begins with the word itself. The noun *resut* (*rsw.t*), attested throughout Pharaonic history, derives from the verbal root *rs* meaning "to awake." The dream is not unconsciousness but heightened vigilance—an awakening into perception unavailable to ordinary waking sight. The scribal convention of classifying *resut* with the hieroglyphic determinative of the "open eye" confirms it.

Unlike the Mesopotamian model, where divine message arrives from entirely outside the sleeper, the Egyptian framework positions the dreamer at a threshold. One "sees a dream"—the grammatical passivity indicates reception rather than authorship. Yet what is received passes through the dreamer's constitutional nature, registering differently depending on inherent type.

### *The Ramesside Dream Book*

The Ramesside Dream Book (*Papyrus Chester Beatty III*, c. 1220 BCE, with origins potentially reaching the Twelfth Dynasty) provides the foundational Egyptian methodology. Each dream image is treated as a "knot" (*ts.t*) requiring systematic untying through three interlocking techniques: phonetic-semantic correspondence (paronomasia), dream polarity (paradoxical inversion of waking valence), and visual punning on hieroglyphic signs.

The manual's visual organization reinforced its interpretive categories through color. The word "BAD" was written in red — the color of Seth, of the desert, of blood and danger — while all other text appeared in black, enabling immediate discrimination between auspicious and ominous at a glance.

### *Constitutional Typology: Horus and Seth*

The Egyptian manual introduces a fundamental division: the "Followers of Horus" and the "Followers of Seth" (Typhonians). This reflects the Egyptian cosmological understanding that the struggle between Horus and Seth—order against chaos, *Maat* against *Isfet*—manifests within the individual human constitution.

The mantic value of any dream depends upon which type the dreamer embodies. Physical markers (red hair, ruddy complexion for Sethian types) and behavioral patterns (quarrelsome disposition, proneness to disruption) indicate alignment. The same dream symbol carries opposite interpretive weight depending on constitutional type.

### *The Four Sons of Horus*

The Demotic dream books of the Ptolemaic period correlate dream animals with specific deities and their anatomical seats within the dreamer's body. "Feeding" an animal in a dream establishes a ritual relationship between dreamer and deity, localizing within the organ protected by the corresponding Son of Horus: Hapy (lungs), Duamutef (stomach), Qebehsenuef (intestines), and Imsety (liver).

This organ mapping marks a turn inward. The external divine message now localizes in the body—a bridge between Mesopotamian externality and Chinese internalization.

## Indian Development

Indian traditions weave dream interpretation into astrological timing and constitutional medicine. The *svapna* doctrine divides the night into watches from dusk to dawn, with dreams in each watch carrying different predictive validity and manifestation timing. Dreams in the first watch have long-range validity; those just before waking manifest immediately.

The Moon's *nakṣatra* placement colors dream significance—the planetary ruler of the lunar mansion shapes interpretation. Saturn dreams during Saturn periods suggest karmic themes; Jupiter dreams during Jupiter transits indicate spiritual advancement or material prosperity. The *doṣa* (constitutional humor) and *guṇa* (quality of nature) frameworks from Āyurveda provide the physiological substrate through which celestial influence registers.

The Indian system stands between poles—dreams carry celestial significance filtered through bodily constitution, with timing protocols assessing validity and manifestation.

## Chinese Medical Oneiromancy

In Classical Chinese Medicine, dreams arise from the condition of the five organ-spirits (*wǔ shén*), with specific dream content revealing the state of corresponding organs. The ethereal soul (*hún*) bears primary responsibility for dream generation—during sleep, it wanders, and its journeys constitute the dream experience.

This is the fully internal model. The sky has been brought inside the body through the Eight Extraordinary Vessels, which serve as internal wiring for celestial influences. The *hún* and *pò* souls—associated with the Azure Dragon of the East and White Tiger of the West—correspond to the same cardinal orientations documented in the Puyang M45 burial (c. 4500 BCE), predating Mesopotamian written records by millennia.

Dream diagnosis reads the movement of *shén* through the *zàng-fǔ* organ systems—not external omen requiring propitiation but internal state requiring medical intervention. The three dedicated chapters on Chinese oneiromancy later in this volume explore these dynamics in clinical depth.

## Greek Development

Homer's assertion that "the dream is from Zeus" established the theological foundation for Greek oneiromancy. Yet the Greeks recognized that not all dreams carry divine significance. Penelope's distinction between the gates of ivory (false dreams) and horn (true dreams) marks an early effort to separate prophetic vision from nocturnal noise.

The Greek carries a pun lost in translation. *Elephas* (ivory) sounds like *elephairomai* (to deceive); *keras* (horn) echoes *kraino* (to fulfill). Homer hid the meaning in the music of the words. The problem of veracity—which dreams can be trusted—became central to Greek development and subsequent systems of practice.

## *The Asclepian Tradition*

The healing sanctuaries of Asclepius developed temple incubation into refined therapeutic art. Pilgrims seeking healing underwent ritual purification, offered sacrifice, and slept in the *abaton* (sacred dormitory) awaiting divine visitation. Asclepius would appear in dreams, either healing the supplicant directly or prescribing treatment for implementation upon waking.

This practice likely included a pharmacological dimension. Opium poppy artifacts appear in the archaeological record; days of fasting lowered the threshold for psychoactive effects. The serpents, the music, the miracle stories read aloud—all primed expectancy. Botanical preparation and ritual setting worked together.

Votive inscriptions at Epidaurus record centuries of encounters. The rhetorician Aelius Aristides documented his decades-long relationship with Asclepius through dreams, recording prescriptions for diet, exercise, bathing, and medical treatment. His *Hieroi Logoi* remains our most intimate account of sustained dream-based medical guidance from antiquity.

## *Artemidorus and Systematic Classification*

Artemidorus of Daldis, writing in the second century CE, produced antiquity's most comprehensive surviving treatment of dream interpretation. His *Oneirocritica* distinguishes *enhypnia*—dreams arising from bodily states like hunger, thirst, or sexual desire—from *oneiroi*, prophetic dreams requiring interpretation.

Artemidorus insisted that dream symbols cannot be interpreted mechanically. The same image means different things depending on the dreamer's profession, social status, health, age, and circumstances. A craftsman dreaming of fire has a different relationship to that element than a physician or sailor. The interpreter must know the dreamer before venturing interpretation—an echo of Egyptian constitutional typology.

### *Macrobius and the Five-Fold Classification*

Macrobius, writing around 400 CE, systematized dream classification in his commentary on Cicero's *Somnium Scipionis*. Drawing on Porphyry's lost work, he identifies five types: *somnium* (enigmatic dream requiring interpretation), *visio* (prophetic vision), *oraculum* (authoritative guidance), *insomnium* (nightmare from bodily or emotional disturbance), and *visum* (hypnagogic hallucination). Only the first three possess prophetic significance.

This schema gave Christian Europe a permission to take dreams seriously while maintaining skepticism. The problem of veracity remained central—a concern medieval systematizers like Bonatti would address through astrological protocols.

### *Neoplatonic Synthesis*

Synesius of Cyrene, writing in the early fifth century CE, emphasized that dreams come to everyone. Unlike divination requiring expensive sacrifices, specialized training, or temple access, dreams come freely each night. The poor farmer receives divine communication as readily as the emperor.

Synesius understood dreams as messages transmitted through the subtle body mediating between intellect and flesh. A soul purified through philosophical practice received clearer transmissions than one clouded by passion. Dream interpretation thus joined the Neoplatonic program of purification and ascent—a framework that would shape both Islamic and Christian reception.

## Comparative Classification Systems

Each tradition developed methods for distinguishing significant dreams from meaningless nocturnal disturbance:

*Table 1.1. Comparative Classification Systems*

| Tradition | Significant Dreams | Meaningless Dreams |
|---|---|---|
| Homer | Gates of Horn (True) | Gates of Ivory (False) |
| Mesopotamian | Divine Message (Zaqīqu) | Demonic Disturbance |
| Egyptian | *Resut (Awakening-Vision)* | *Dw rsw.t (Nightmare/Attack)* |
| Artemidorus | *Oneiroi (Prophetic)* | *Enhypnia (Somatic)* |
| Macrobius | *Somnium, Visio, Oraculum* | *Insomnium, Visum* |
| Vedic | First/Second Watch Dreams | Third Watch Dreams |
| Chinese | *Shén Movement (Organ-Spirit)* | Pathological Disturbance |

# The External-Internal Spectrum

The oneiromantic traditions map along a spectrum from fully external (divine message requiring outward ritual response) to fully internal (organ-spirit condition requiring medical intervention):

*Table 1.2. The External-Internal Spectrum*

| Tradition | Dream Source | Interpretation Mode | Remediation |
|---|---|---|---|
| Mesopotamian | External (Zaqīqu) | Ominal (State Fate) | *Namburbi (Apotropaic Ritual)* |
| Egyptian | Threshold (Liminal) | Constitutional | Ritual + Organ Attention |
| Indian | Celestial-Karmic | *Doṣa/Guṇa Mediated* | Timing + Propitiation |
| Greek | Divine/ Somatic Mixed | Context-Dependent | Incubation + Medicine |
| Chinese | *Internal (Hún/Pò)* | *Zàng-Fǔ Diagnostic* | Medical Intervention |

## Toward a Celestial Synthesis

Not all dreams matter equally. Distinguishing the significant from the trivial remains essential across all traditions. Interpreters must know both symbolic vocabulary and the dreamer's circumstances. Threatening dreams need not manifest when ritual, medical, or spiritual measures address their causes.

The celestial dimension grounds subjective imagery in objective pattern. Relevant charts include the consultation chart, the moment of the dream, or the moment of recollection. The natal chart reveals the dreamer's characteristic receptivity to prophetic experience; the horary yields specific prediction for the dream at hand.

### *The Ninth House as Prophetic Locus*

The ninth house—the *Domus Dei,* House of God—governs prophecy, divination, higher knowledge, and dream interpretation. Its condition describes whether a dream carries portent. The ninth lord's essential dignity indicates whether the dream speaks true: elevated dignity suggests a dream worthy of interpretation; peregrine or debilitated warns of phantasm from bodily disturbance or emotional residue.

A career dream might prove false if the ninth lord is peregrine. A trivial dream might prove significant if the ninth lord is dignified and well-aspected by benefics. Content and veracity are distinct: the ninth house ruler and planets therein govern what the dream concerns; essential dignity and aspect determine whether to trust it.

### *Timing and the Tripartite Night*

In clinical practice, the night divides into three phases, each serving different function. The first third processes the day's experiences—sorting, consolidating, managing mundane material. The middle third opens into prophetic territory where divinatory content becomes accessible. The final third reorganizes the psyche for the coming day.

This tripartite structure maps onto the triplicity lords governing each elemental sign—the same pattern operating across a lifetime and within a single night. The Vedic system similarly emphasizes timing: dreams in the first watch have the longest predictive range; those in the final watch may manifest within days. Integrating Western triplicity doctrine with Vedic watch-timing provides precise tools for assessing when to attend most closely and how long manifestation may require.

## The Chapters Ahead

The dream is old. Before psychology named it, before neuroscience mapped it, the ancients read it—as omen, as oracle, as letter from the gods. Mesopotamian scribes catalogued its grammar. Egyptian priests decoded its constitutional signatures. Greek pilgrims slept in temple darkness awaiting its cure. Chinese physicians diagnosed organ-spirit wandering through its imagery. The methods differed; the recognition did not. What arrives in sleep carries meaning. The art lies in discerning what kind.

Chapter Two examines dreams as vehicles of communal law and healing in non-literate traditions. Chapters Three and Four present Mesopotamian and Egyptian systems—the *Iškar Zaqīqu*, the *āšipu*'s ritual repertoire, Gula's somatic dimension, the *ts.t* protocol, Horus/Seth constitutional typology, the Four Sons organ mapping. Chapter Five explores the Indian *svapna* doctrine with its timing protocols and *nakṣatra* correlations.

Chapters Six through Eight present Chinese medical oneiromancy in the detail its clinical importance warrants—*hún/pò* dynamics, Five *Shén* organ correlations, diagnostic methodology. Chapters Ten through Twelve trace the Western synthesis from Greece through Persia and Arabia to Bonatti's medieval protocols for judging dream veracity. Chapter Thirteen provides syncretic integration for clinical navigation across systems. Chapter Fourteen addresses botanical allies for dream work.

The pan-celestial framework established in the *History and Foundations* volume comes to clinical ground here. Each tradition accessed the same sky; each developed distinctive methods for reading its nightly inscription upon the human soul. The practitioner who understands all positions along this spectrum commands the full range of what celestial oneiromancy offers.

# Sources


Aristides, Aelius. *Hieroi Logoi (Sacred Tales)*. Translated by C. A. Behr. Leiden: Brill, 1968.

Artemidorus of Daldis. *Oneirocritica*. Translated by Robert J. White. Park Ridge, NJ: Noyes Press, 1975.

Butler, Sally A. L. *Mesopotamian Conceptions of Dreams and Dream Rituals*. Münster: Ugarit-Verlag, 1998.

Edelstein, Emma J., and Ludwig Edelstein. *Asclepius: Collection and Interpretation of the Testimonies*. 2 vols. Baltimore: Johns Hopkins University Press, 1945.

Gardiner, Alan H. *Hieratic Papyri in the British Museum, Third Series: Chester Beatty Gift*. 2 vols. London: British Museum, 1935.

Homer. *Iliad*. Translated by Richmond Lattimore. Chicago: University of Chicago Press, 1951.

Homer. *Odyssey*. Translated by Richmond Lattimore. New York: Harper & Row, 1965.

*Huangdi Neijing Lingshu* (Spiritual Pivot). In *Huangdi Neijing*. Compiled ca. 1st century BCE.

Macrobius. *Commentary on the Dream of Scipio*. Translated by William Harris Stahl. New York: Columbia University Press, 1952.

Oppenheim, A. Leo. "The Interpretation of Dreams in the Ancient Near East." *Transactions of the American Philosophical Society* 46, no. 3 (1956): 179–373.

Rochberg, Francesca. *The Heavenly Writing: Divination, Horoscopy, and Astronomy in Mesopotamian Culture*. Cambridge: Cambridge University Press, 2004.

Szpakowska, Kasia. *Behind Closed Eyes: Dreams and Nightmares in Ancient Egypt*. Swansea: Classical Press of Wales, 2003.

Synesius of Cyrene. *On Dreams*. Translated by Isaac Myer. Philadelphia, 1888.

Varahamihira. *Bṛhat Saṃhitā*. Translated by M. Ramakrishna Bhat. Delhi: Motilal Banarsidass, 1981.

## Chapter Two

# Dreams as Communal Law and Healing

*ἴδιος κόσμος ἐστὶν ὁ τῶν ἐγρηγορότων· τῶν δὲ κοιμωμένων ἕκαστος εἰς ἴδιον ἀποστρέφεται*

*"The waking have one common world, but the sleeping turn aside each into a world of his own."*

—Heraclitus, Fragment B89

# The Ropes Descend

The afternoon I received the Rod of Asclepius tattoo, Bradford Keeney arrived in San Francisco.

My team was marking a threshold—my cohort at CIIS moving into dissertation approval, the formal recognition that our scholarly work had found its direction. The single serpent wound around the staff seemed fitting: the god of healing, the snake that sheds its skin and emerges renewed, the vertical axis connecting earth to the hand that holds it. Asclepius was the wounded healer, son of Apollo, raised by Chiron—killed by Zeus for raising the dead, then placed among the stars as Ophiuchus, the Serpent-Bearer. I did not yet understand what I was inscribing on my body. The rod marks healing through transformation, the physician who has himself been broken and remade. I was marking myself for a death I did not know was coming.

Keeney was in town for an intensive. He had spent decades with the Ju/'hoansi of the Kalahari, receiving initiation into the healing ways of the San—the oldest continuous human culture, carrying practices that predate the separation of tribes, the emergence of agriculture, perhaps the differentiation of language itself. The San distinguish between two domains of existence. The First Creation—ǂain ǂaingǂani—is the original state: pre-linguistic, fluid, undifferentiated wholeness where everything constantly changes form. The Second Creation—g!xoa—is the world we inhabit: the realm of stable names, fixed identities, the separations that language creates. In the First Creation, there was no death, no sickness. The "great turning around" occurred when animals and people were given names, freezing them into bounded forms. Healing, in San understanding, means crossing the border back into the First Creation to re-infuse the community with the vital changing force. This crossing requires the dissolution of Second Creation structures—including the structure of the self.

When San healers dance, they draw down n/om—spiritual energy, the same force other traditions call qì or prāṇa—until their bodies shake uncontrollably and their spirits slip out of their skins to travel where healing is needed. The shaking is not symptom but vehicle. It is the body's way of surrendering Second Creation coherence so that First Creation power can move through.

At the gathering the next evening, surrounded by cohort members in our second year of the program, Keeney transferred the shaking. The ropes to God descended. N/om entered my body—not as metaphor but as current, as fire, as the trembling that dissolves the boundary between what I am and what I serve.

I had practiced medicine for decades by then. I had studied pulse diagnosis with masters, learned the classical formulary, treated thousands of patients with acupuncture and herbs. All of this was Second Creation work: learning a system of names, applying categories to conditions, balancing what could be labeled. I thought I understood what healing meant. But when the shaking entered me, my mission changed. The phrase I had carried for years—"enculturating Chinese medicine in the West"—fell away. That phrase belonged to the Second Creation: teaching a tradition, translating a system, fitting ancient wisdom into modern institutional forms. What remained was simpler and more demanding: deep personal and collective transformation. First Creation work. The dreams that followed showed me what that meant.

The Rod of Asclepius I had inscribed that afternoon suddenly made sense. The serpent sheds its skin—the old form dies so the new can emerge. The wounded healer knows illness from the inside. Asclepius himself died and was reborn as a constellation, the Serpent-Bearer holding his snake across the ecliptic, the thirteenth sign that disrupts the tidy twelve. I had marked my body for border crossing before I knew the border existed.

This is how communal dream traditions work. Not information assembled from ethnographic distance, but transmission that reorganizes the receiver. The dream is not private. The vision is not yours to keep. What you receive, you carry for others.

## The Social Body of the Dream

Heraclitus observed that sleepers turn aside into private worlds. The modern West agrees: dreams are individual psychological events, symptoms of personal history, accessible only to the dreamer and perhaps an analyst. This privatization of dream life is historically anomalous. Communal dream traditions—where dreams carry public weight, demand social interpretation, and generate collective obligation—are the human norm. The dream-sharing circle preceded the analyst's couch by millennia.

In oral societies, the boundary between waking and dreaming is porous or absent. For the Yanomami of the Amazon basin, waking life and dreamed life carry equivalent ontological weight. When a person dreams, the body remains in the hammock while the pei utupë—the soul-image—detaches and travels. It encounters relatives living and deceased; the experiences it gathers are events that have already occurred or potential realities capable of affecting the entire community. The dream is empirical knowledge, a distinct channel for accessing information, solving problems, understanding the self in relation to the collective.

These traditions do not separate the dream world from the celestial world. The same sky that regulates seasons, marks time, and provides navigational guidance governs dream life. Stars signal when to seek visions; lunar phases determine when dreams carry prophetic weight; celestial bodies appear within dreams as messengers. Before literate civilizations systematized the connection into formal astrology, oral cultures recognized that the heavens and the dreaming mind participate in a single cosmic order. This chapter surveys these traditions to establish that celestial and oneiric knowledge—the foundation of astrological oneiromancy—emerges from humanity's oldest ways of understanding the night.

On the spectrum running from external to internal—from dreams received as divine message to dreams arising from bodily condition—communal traditions occupy territory near the external pole, but with a distinctive social dimension absent from later literate developments. The dream arrives from outside the individual: ancestors, spirits, the Dreaming itself. Yet the response it demands is collective rather than private. Where Mesopotamian priests performed apotropaic ritual and Chinese physicians prescribed herbal formulae, oral cultures mobilized the community. The Haudenosaunee assembled to fulfill a dream's demands; the San danced together to metabolize what the healer had seen. External source, communal remedy. The dream belongs to the group before it belongs to the dreamer.

# Tjukurrpa: The Aboriginal Australian Dreaming

The Aboriginal Australian concept of the Dreaming (Tjukurrpa in Western Desert languages, Alcheringa or Jukurrpa in other language groups) is the most comprehensive integration of dream consciousness with social organization, territorial relationship, and celestial observation found anywhere on earth. W.E.H. Stanner showed that the Dreaming is not a past era—not a mythic "once upon a time"—but an eternal present underlying ordinary reality. The ancestral beings who shaped the land during the creation period did not disappear; their spiritual essence, or guruwari, remains active within the landscape and the night sky alike. Sacred sites on earth mirror sacred patterns in the heavens. To know one is to know both.

## *Songlines, Sacred Geography, and the Stellar Map*

Songlines crisscross the Australian continent, encoding narrative and navigation. Deborah Bird Rose documents how an initiated person can "sing" their way across hundreds of miles of unfamiliar territory, following verses that describe an ancestral being's journey. Each verse corresponds to geographic features—waterhole, rock formation, tree—created or encountered during the Dreaming. The songlines are not confined to earth. The Wardaman of Northern Australia describe "Dark Sparklers"—celestial songlines mirroring terrestrial ones, where stars serve as a compass and mnemonic for the land below.

This integration of terrestrial and celestial geography carries legal force. Wardaman tradition prescribes sleeping with the head oriented eastward, aligned with the sun's rising path. To sleep westward—toward the setting sun—violates natural order. The sleeping body participates in cosmic alignment. Even the position of the dreamer's head falls under celestial law.

## *The Emu in the Sky: Stellar Timing and Resource Law*

A defining feature of Australian ethnoastronomy is the recognition of dark nebulae—opaque clouds of interstellar dust blocking the Milky Way's light—as significant constellations. Where Western astronomy sees absence, Aboriginal astronomers see presence: shape formed by darkness against the river of stars. The most prominent of these dark constellations is the Emu in the Sky, whose head is the Coalsack Nebula near the Southern Cross, body extending along the Great Rift into Scorpius.

The celestial emu's orientation throughout the year provides a biological and legal calendar. When it reaches a specific angle in the evening sky—appearing to run along the horizon—terrestrial emus are laying eggs. This is the time to harvest, ensuring resources are taken at peak availability in accordance with environmental law encoded in the stars. The celestial emu does not merely symbolize the earthly bird; it governs human interaction with that bird through legally binding astronomical timing.

## *The Seven Sisters and Kinship Jurisprudence*

The Pleiades—called the Seven Sisters across Aboriginal Australia—carries one of the most widespread and legally significant Dreaming narratives. Seven sisters flee across the land and eventually into the sky, pursued by a male figure (often associated with Orion) who belongs to an inappropriate kinship category. In Warlpiri tradition, the sisters belong to the Napaljarri skin group, and the pursuing man violates marriage law by his pursuit.

This celestial drama is not myth but active jurisprudence. The narrative is enacted during Kurdiji initiation ceremonies, where young men learn the laws of the community at sites like Yanjirlypirri ("star place"). The stars serve as eternal witnesses to the legal order established in the Dreaming. When the Pleiades rise in the pre-dawn sky, they announce the season; when they feature in dreams, they invoke the kinship laws they eternally embody. The dreamer who encounters the Seven Sisters receives not personal symbolism but legal instruction.

## *Dream Validation and Cultural Innovation*

Individuals access the Dreaming directly through sleep. A person may receive in nocturnal vision a song, a ceremonial design, or knowledge of a country previously unknown to them. These special night dreams are not automatically credited; elders determine whether the dream genuinely connects to Dreaming reality or represents personal fantasy. Validated dreams enter collective heritage and may be transmitted across generations.

Among the Mardu and other Western Desert groups, the dream spirit or eye soul (partunjarri) detaches from the body during sleep to travel and gather revelations. These journeys are as true as physical travel, allowing individuals to visit homelands, check on kin, or encounter ancestors—including stellar ancestors who dwell in the night sky. Artists and singers frequently receive new material through dreams: mythological images, ceremonial forms, healing songs. These dream-received rituals, partunjarrijanu, serve as cultural capital and function as currency in regional exchange between tribes. The dream connects the individual to the cosmic order mapped in land and sky alike.

## The Kalahari San: Fire in the Spine and the Singing Stars

The San traditions carry weight for this work that the other surveys do not. What follows requires a different voice. I have standing here—not the standing of a Ju/'hoan elder, never that, but the standing of someone whose body has been reorganized by practice.

Among the Ju/'hoansi, dreams serve as the primary vehicle through which healers receive power. The central practice—the all-night trance dance—mobilizes n/om through rhythmic singing, clapping, and movement until healers enter !kia, the altered state in which healing occurs. The songs powering these dances come through dreams. The dreams connect with the stars.

N/om lives at the base of the spine and belly, "sleeping" until awakened. The San describe "boiling energy": communal singing generates spiritual heat, activating an "internal pump" that pushes energy up through the spine into the head, producing spontaneous shaking. The first time it rose in me, I understood why they call it fire—not warmth but burning, the spine a column of heat, the skull a pressure demanding release. The trembling begins without volition. I had practiced qìgōng for years; this was different. The shaking came from elsewhere, doing what it needed with or without my cooperation. What was required was surrender.

When n/om reaches the skull, the healer's spirit "slips out of its skin"—the moment of !kia where healing occurs, where contact with ancestors becomes possible. The same pathway operates in dream: the dream-body travels to stellar realms, receives instruction, returns with gifts. Sleep, trance, stellar connection—three access points to a single territory.

The Ju/'hoan tradition maps development through stations. What Keeney transferred that night moved me into Station Three work, where the healer transmits "nails" of energy through the hands. The languaging of my mission changed because the cognitive mind was no longer directing. Words give way to music. The practitioner becomes instrument rather than agent.

San healers speak of a "rope to God" (n!uan-tso) that pulls them toward the spirit realm—tangible, kinesthetic reality connecting the healer to the Sky God, source of n/om. Horizontal ropes also connect the community, belly button to belly button. The San say this is their true government—organized around maintenance of spiritual heat rather than political power. Dreams arrive along these ropes: not psychological events but deliveries from where healing power originates.

The Ju/'hoansi believe the stars "sing loudly"—the night sky resonant with power. The music of the healing dance channels stellar music. Canopus serves as winter marker; Sirius is the "Grandmother of Canopus." The Southern Cross and Pointers are lions, once people before transformation. Not metaphors but cosmological facts: stars are ancestors, their positions governing ritual timing and dreams received.

San mythology tells how stars came to be: a celestial ostrich flew across an unlit world, dropping glowing feathers. The final feather blazed so bright it became the moon. The scattered feathers became stars. This image grounds the work when celestial medicine risks becoming another system to master. The stars glow because something living dropped them there.

When I received the shaking, I received an obligation. The n/om does not belong to me. It moves through me toward wherever needed. The dreamer is not a composer but a receiver, and having received, must give. This changes how I understand clinical work. The patient bringing a dream is reporting a transmission. Something came through. Our work is to understand what arrived and what it requires.

## The Haudenosaunee: Oracle of the Soul and the Pleiades Zenith

The Haudenosaunee (Iroquois) Confederacy maintains one of the most rigorous dream traditions in North America, its timing governed by astronomical observation. Seventeenth-century Jesuit accounts document that for the Iroquois and neighboring Huron, the dream was the "principal Divinity"—an oracle to be followed with exactness. Their dream work centers on the belief that the soul possesses desires (ondinnonk) distinct from the conscious mind's agendas. These hidden desires express themselves through dream language; if left unsatisfied, the soul may become "angry," leading to physical illness, mental disturbance, or the catastrophic condition of soul loss.

### *The Pleiades Zenith and the Lunar Trigger*

The most significant Haudenosaunee dream work occurs during the Midwinter Ceremony—the nine-day New Year's festival of comprehensive renewal. Timing is determined not by a static calendar but by astronomical observation. Faithkeepers track the Pleiades as it dominates the winter sky. When the cluster reaches zenith at dusk, the astronomical precondition is met.

The stellar signal alone is not sufficient. After the Pleiades zenith, the community waits for the first new moon of the year. The ceremony begins five days later. This dual requirement—stellar position plus lunar phase—synchronizes communal renewal with both sidereal and synodic cycles. The Midwinter Ceremony sits at the intersection of stellar time and lunar time, weaving psychological renewal into celestial order.

### *The Ononharoia: Dream Guessing Rite*

The Ononharoia, or Dream Guessing Rite, is a public event where community members attempt to unriddle the dreams of those troubled by them, protecting dreamers from the obsession generated by unfulfilled soul desires. The process is structured. An individual troubled by dreams goes from house to house searching for someone capable of guessing the dream's content. Community members exert intuition to identify the hidden wish. The dreamer provides feedback only through affirmative or negative responses until the correct desire is identified.

Once guessed, the community becomes obligated to help fulfill the dream's command—providing a specific object, hosting a feast, or performing a particular action. The therapeutic burden is distributed across the collective; no individual bears the weight of their soul's demands alone. The timing—governed by Pleiades and moon—ensures this communal dream work occurs when celestial conditions support psychological transformation.

### *Medicine Societies and Soul Recovery*

When dreams cause mental or physical symptoms, medicine societies conduct curing ceremonies. The False Face Society performs exorcisms in carved masks, house to house, frightening away disease spirits and fulfilling dream requirements. The atetshents—"one who dreams"—is a doctor, a shaman. These specialists take a piece of the patient's clothing, wrap tobacco in it, and sleep with it to receive a diagnostic dream. Dreams determine causes and cures—not symptoms but diagnostic instruments. Fail to heed repeated warnings, risk soul loss: the free soul abandons the body, leaving a mechanical being, one of the walking dead.

## The Achuar: Tactical Intelligence and the Morning Star

In the Amazonian rainforests of Ecuador and Peru, the Achuar and related Shuar peoples maintain a daily dream-sharing ritual that serves as the cornerstone of social and tactical existence. The Achuar equate reality with dreaming, believing the soul departs the body during sleep to enter the real from which waking life derives. Dreams are not reflections of waking life but its foundation. Their relationship with Venus—the Morning Star—structures both dream practice and strategic worldview.

## *Venus as Tactical Guide*

The Achuar have historically been a warrior culture; their relationship with the Morning Star is tied to this identity. Venus, appearing for approximately 236 days as morning star before disappearing and reappearing as evening star, mirrors tactical patterns of ambush, retreat, and return that characterize Amazonian warfare. The planet's visibility cycle provides a strategic framework: when Venus blazes in the pre-dawn sky, it signals assertive action; disappearance signals withdrawal and concealment.

This astronomical lore extends to dream interpretation. Dreams received when Venus is prominent as Morning Star carry a different weight than dreams received during its absence or evening star phase. Dream interpreters factor planetary visibility into the assessment of what a dream means and how the community should respond. In the 1990s, Achuar elders saw the threat of oil development in their dreams before it arrived physically, allowing them to organize a unified political front to protect their territory—tactical intelligence delivered through dreams, validated against celestial signs.

## *The Hora de Wayusa*

The Achuar day begins between 3:00 and 4:00 AM with the hora de wayusa. Families gather around a communal fire to drink wayusa, a caffeinated tea brewed from Ilex guayusa, a shade-grown holly. The caffeine heightens focus and memory during dream-sharing. Women gather, dry, and boil the leaves overnight so the infusion is ready before dawn—the hour when Venus, if visible, stands brightest in the eastern sky.

Participants drink several bowls, then induce vomiting as physical and spiritual purification. Families sit together; each member recounts the night's dreams. The household elder interprets, piecing together information from collective dreams to navigate the day. Dreams provide tactical guidance: where the game will be found, which paths are dangerous, what conflicts require attention, whether planned activities should proceed or be abandoned. The pre-dawn timing ensures interpretation occurs while the stellar and planetary configuration of the night remains visible—the same sky that presided over the dreams can be consulted during their interpretation.

### Future Alteration

The Achuar are not fatalistic. If a negative event is foreseen, they take corrective steps. The dream reveals trajectory, not fate. For significant threats, shamans use ayahuasca or maikua (Brugmansia) to induce deeper visionary states aimed at dream exchange or future alteration. Children are taught to move toward dream threats; grasp the threat, conquer fear, and the frightening vision collapses to reveal its true message.

## The Temiar: Spirit Songs from the Resonant Landscape

The dream practices of the Temiar of the Malaysian rainforest center on a reciprocal relationship between the dreamer and the spirits of their environment. In Temiar cosmology, the head soul travels during sleep and encounters the souls of other entities—plants, animals, geographic features like mountains or rivers. Marina Roseman's ethnomusicological fieldwork documents how these encounters generate the ceremonial songs that structure Temiar healing and social life.

These songs are performed in ceremonies timed to seasonal cycles—fruiting of trees, flowering of plants, and astronomical markers indicating transition. The dreamer-medium sings the phrases received in a dream. A chorus of women and girls repeats them, providing percussive accompaniment with bamboo-tube stampers (go:h) beaten against a log. The ceremonies maintain cosmic order and treat soul loss.

The Temiar position the landscape as musically animate—every tree, river, mountain possesses a soul capable of teaching songs. The dream is a site of interspecies communication where boundaries between human and nonhuman dissolve into shared melody. The forest sings through human voices; humans receive instruction from vegetal and mineral teachers. The dream opens a channel that waking consciousness cannot access, allowing the more-than-human world to participate in human cultural production.

Jon Hassell's *Dream Theory in Malaya*, drawing on Kilton Stewart's Senoi fieldwork in this region, brought this material into contemporary musical practice and influenced my own work in sound healing—another instance where scholarly study and embodied practice refused to remain separate.

## Hebrew Prophetic Dreams: Celestial Sovereignty

The Hebrew scriptures preserve a complex tradition of prophetic dreaming in which celestial imagery carries political and theological weight. Jacob's dream at Bethel—the ladder with angels ascending and descending, the divine voice promising land and descendants—establishes the pattern: dream as a site of covenant encounter, geographic location becoming sacred through nocturnal revelation.

### *Joseph's Celestial Dream and Tribal Sovereignty*

Joseph's second dream in Genesis 37 introduces explicitly astronomical symbolism: "Behold, I have dreamed yet another dream: and behold, the sun and the moon and eleven stars bowed down to me." Jacob immediately interprets the celestial bodies: the sun represents Jacob himself, the moon Rachel, and the eleven stars Joseph's brothers. The dream provokes fraternal jealousy leading to Joseph's enslavement—yet its fulfillment, when his family bows before him in Egypt, validates the prophetic vision.

Later Jewish tradition connected the twelve tribes to the zodiac. The tribes arranged around the Tabernacle correspond to the four fixed signs: Judah east as Lion, Ephraim west as Bull, Reuben south as Man, Dan north as Eagle (substituting for Scorpion). Israel becomes a terrestrial reflection of celestial order—each tribe holding jurisdiction modeled on the stars. Joseph's dream of celestial prostration is not family drama but cosmological sovereignty: the zodiac itself acknowledges his authority.

### *Prophetic Hierarchy and Communal Consequence*

Numbers 12:6 establishes a hierarchy: "If there be a prophet among you, I the Lord will make myself known unto him in a vision, and will speak unto him in a dream." Dreams are one tier of prophetic reception—not the highest (Moses spoke with God "mouth to mouth"), but legitimate. Joel promises that in the last days, "your old men shall dream dreams, your young men shall see visions"—prophetic access democratized beyond the institutional office.

Prophetic dreams carry social consequences. Joseph's interpretations determine state policy on grain storage; Daniel's visions concern the fate of empires. Celestial symbolism in these dreams—suns, moons, stars—is not decorative but jurisdictional. When heavenly bodies appear in prophetic vision, they invoke the cosmic order governing earthly kingdoms. The dream may be received individually; its celestial content signals transpersonal significance.

## The Vision Quest: Stellar Orientation and Communal Validation

Across North American Indigenous cultures, the vision quest (hanbleceya in Lakota, "crying for a vision") represents a formalized practice for seeking a dream vision under specific celestial conditions. The seeker withdraws to an isolated location—hilltop, forest clearing, sacred site—and remains without food or water for four days and nights. Deprivation and solitude thin the veil between ordinary and visionary consciousness, creating conditions in which guardian spirits may appear.

Timing and orientation are not arbitrary. The seeker begins at a significant astronomical moment—solstice, equinox, or particular lunar phase. The vision space is oriented to the cardinal directions, aligning the seeker's body with the solar path and celestial poles. Among Plains tribes, the seeker faces east to greet the rising sun; the four days correspond to the four directions, the four seasons, and the four phases of the moon. The vision sought is not personal insight but alignment with cosmic order.

Preparation involves guidance from elders who determine readiness and timing based on the individual's condition and celestial factors. Upon returning, the seeker recounts the vision to elders who interpret its meaning and determine its implications for the community's role. A vision may reveal a calling as healer, warrior, or ceremonial leader; it may provide a new name, a song, or specific instructions for life conduct. Preparation, reception, integration—the tripartite structure ensures celestial timing, visionary content, and communal validation work together.

## The Communal Function of Dreams: A Synthesis

These traditions converge on principles that challenge modern Western assumptions—and establish the foundation for astrological oneiromancy.

Dreams carry public weight. A dream is not the dreamer's private experience but potentially affects the family, community, and territory. The Aboriginal dreamer who receives a song, the Achuar hunter who dreams of game, the Haudenosaunee patient whose unfulfilled dream produces illness—all demonstrate that dreams shape collective reality.

Interpretation requires community. The elder who decodes the Achuar family's morning dreams, the Haudenosaunee neighbor who guesses the soul's hidden desire, the Temiar chorus who performs the dreamer's spirit song—meaning emerges through social process, not solitary reflection. The dream speaks in symbolic language, but the dictionary is held collectively.

Dreams generate obligation. A dream received carries responsibilities—ritual fulfillment, public announcement, and therapeutic application. To dream is to become answerable: to the community that must satisfy soul demands, to the spirits who transmitted the vision, to the ancestors whose knowledge requires transmission.

Dreams and stars participate in a single cosmic order. The Aboriginal Emu in the Sky governs when terrestrial emu eggs may be harvested;

the Haudenosaunee Pleiades zenith triggers communal dream work; the Achuar Morning Star shapes tactical interpretation; the San draw healing power from singing stars; Joseph's celestial dream establishes tribal sovereignty. Not isolated instances but expressions of universal recognition: the powers governing the heavens govern the dreaming mind. The sky is not the backdrop to dream life but its regulator and source.

*Table 2.1: Celestial Elements in Communal Dream Traditions*

| Tradition | Celestial Marker | Dream Function | Integration |
|---|---|---|---|
| Aboriginal Australian | Emu in the Sky (Coalsack); Pleiades (Seven Sisters); dark nebulae | Resource timing; kinship law; navigation | Songlines mirror stellar paths; validated dreams enter Law |
| Kalahari San | Canopus (winter marker); Sirius; Southern Cross; 'singing stars' | Healing power; seasonal ritual timing | Stars provide n/om; healers travel to stellar realms |
| Haudenosaunee | Pleiades zenith; lunar phases (new moon) | Midwinter timing; soul restoration | Stellar + lunar conjunction triggers ceremony |
| Achuar/Shuar | Venus (Morning Star); pre-dawn sky | Tactical guidance; future alteration | Planetary visibility affects dream interpretation |
| Hebrew Prophetic | Sun, Moon, stars (zodiacal); tribal-stellar mapping | Sovereignty; state policy; eschatology | Celestial prostration = political authority |
| Vision Quest | Cardinal directions; solstice/equinox; lunar phase | Life calling; guardian spirit contact | Celestial timing + orientation govern quest |

# The Question the Oral Traditions Leave Us

The literate civilizations that follow in subsequent chapters—Mesopotamia, Egypt, Greece, India, China—systematized the connection between stars and dreams into protocols that could be recorded, transmitted, and refined across generations. What they added was invaluable: the accumulation of observation, the correlation of images with outcomes, the development of techniques teachable beyond a single lineage.

## What Was Lost

But they also lost something.

The oral traditions know that dreams belong to communities before they belong to individuals. The Haudenosaunee mobilize the entire village to fulfill a troubling dream's demands. The San dance together to metabolize what the healer has seen. The Achuar family gathers at 3 AM to piece together what the night has delivered. No one faces their dreams alone.

The contemporary clinician works differently. The patient arrives individually, reports a dream, and departs. The therapeutic dyad has replaced the village. The analyst's couch has replaced the circle around the fire. We have gained privacy and perhaps depth; we have lost the collective that distributes the weight of what dreams demand.

What would it mean to recover something of the communal dimension? Not to abandon the insights of individual psychology—the dream speaks to and of the dreamer—but to remember that some dreams concern family, ancestry, collective fate. When a patient dreams of their dead grandfather, they may be working through personal grief. They may also be receiving a transmission that concerns everyone who shares that bloodline. When a patient dreams of an ecological catastrophe, they may be processing anxiety about the news. They may also be participating in something the entire community needs to metabolize.

The oral traditions would ask: Who else needs to hear this dream? Whose interpretation should be sought? What obligation does the dream generate beyond the dreamer's own integration?

These questions have no simple answers in contemporary practice. The village does not exist in the same form. Professional boundaries constrain who participates in a patient's care. The confidentiality that protects privacy also isolates.

But the questions remain. The dream arrives already embedded in a relationship. Something came through. Our work is to understand what arrived and what it requires—not just for the individual in the room, but for the network of relationship that individual carries.

The fire in the spine does not burn for one person. The ropes descend for anyone willing to climb them. The stars sing whether or not we have ears to hear.

## Practitioner's Inheritance

The clinician stands in this lineage.

Dreams arrive already embedded in relationship. The patient reporting a dream participates in an ancient transaction—vision received, interpretation sought, obligation generated. The clinical encounter remains a dream-sharing circle of two. Receive a dream, become responsible for helping it find meaning.

Timing matters. These cultures did not interpret dreams apart from celestial conditions. The Haudenosaunee waited for the Pleiades and the moon to align. The Achuar factored Venus's visibility. The vision quest began at the solstice or the equinox. For contemporary practice, this translates directly: note the lunar phase when the dream occurred, the planetary hour, and the transits active to the patient's nativity. A dream under Saturn's hour differs from one under Venus's. A dream on a dark moon differs from one at full.

Dreams generate obligation. The Haudenosaunee community was bound to help fulfill the soul's demands. The San healer who received a dream-song had to use it. The clinician who hears a significant dream cannot simply record and move on. Something is owed: attention, interpretation, perhaps action.

Celestial imagery invokes cosmic jurisdiction. When Joseph dreamed of sun, moon, and stars bowing, he dreamed of his place in an order larger than family. When a patient dreams of planets, eclipses, conjunctions—the dream speaks not of personal psychology alone but of the dreamer's relationship to powers governing time itself. Such dreams demand astrological analysis.

The night sky and the dreaming mind speak one language. Learning to read both is the work of celestial medicine.

## Notes

For African dream medicine—particularly Zulu and Xhosa use of Ubulawu (*Silene capensis* and related species)—see Chapter Fourteen: *Oneirobotany*, which provides preparation methods, dosing protocols, and integration with Sangoma divination practice.

## Sources

Descola, Philippe. *The Spears of Twilight: Life and Death in the Amazon Jungle*. Translated by Janet Lloyd. New York: The New Press, 1996.

Hamacher, Duane W., and Ray P. Norris. 'Australian Aboriginal Astronomy: Overview.' *Proceedings of the International Astronomical Union* 7 (2011): 39–47.

Hassell, Jon. *Dream Theory in Malaya*. Editions EG, 1981.

Keeney, Bradford. *Ropes to God: Experiencing the Bushman Spiritual Universe*. Philadelphia: Ringing Rocks Press, 2003.

Keeney, Bradford, and Hillary Keeney. *Way of the Bushman: Spiritual Teachings and Practices of the Kalahari Ju/'hoansi*. Rochester, VT: Bear & Company, 2015.

Norris, Ray P., and Duane W. Hamacher. *Emu Dreaming: An Introduction to Australian Aboriginal Astronomy*. Sydney: Emu Dreaming, 2014.

Rose, Deborah Bird. *Nourishing Terrains: Australian Aboriginal Views of Landscape and Wilderness*. Canberra: Australian Heritage Commission, 1996.

Roseman, Marina. *Healing Sounds from the Malaysian Rainforest: Temiar Music and Medicine*. Berkeley: University of California Press, 1991.

Snodgrass, Mary Ellen. *Encyclopedia of the Literature of Empire*. New York: Facts on File, 2010.

Stanner, W. E. H. *The Dreaming and Other Essays*. Melbourne: Black Inc. Agenda, 2009.

Tedlock, Barbara, ed. *Dreaming: Anthropological and Psychological Interpretations*. Cambridge: Cambridge University Press, 1987.

Wallace, Anthony F. C. 'Dreams and the Wishes of the Soul: A Type of Psychoanalytic Theory Among the Seventeenth Century Iroquois.' *American Anthropologist* 60, no. 2 (1958): 234–248.

Part Two

# Cultural Transmissions

*šiṭir šamê*

**"The writing of heaven."**

—Mesopotamian astronomical term

Nine traditions. Nine ways of reading what the night inscribes.

The chapters that follow trace oneiromancy through its major cultural transmissions: Mesopotamian court science, Egyptian threshold consciousness, Vedic karmic timing, Classical Chinese organ-spirit diagnostics, Daoist sleep cultivation, Tibetan bardo preparation, Greek philosophical synthesis, and the Persian-Arabic methods that would shape medieval Europe.

Each tradition developed sophisticated technology for working with dreams. Each recognized celestial governance over what sleep delivers. Their differences matter—the Mesopotamian *āšipu* and the Chinese physician operate from distinct cosmologies. But their convergences matter more: across millennia and continents, practitioners observed the same sky and the same dreaming mind, and reached overlapping conclusions about their relationship.

What the ancients called *šiṭir šamê*—the writing of heaven—they found inscribed in both domains.

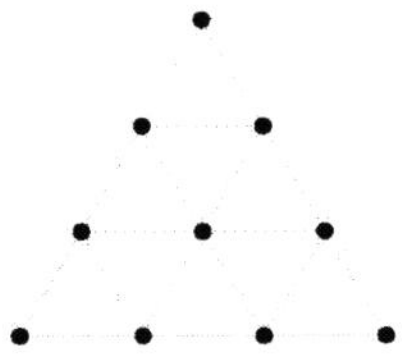

## Chapter Three

# Mesopotamian Oneiromancy

*šiṭir šamê ša ilāni rabûti*

*"The heavenly writing of the great gods"*

—Enūma Anu Enlil

## The External Pole

Mesopotamian civilization produced the oldest surviving written records of systematic dream interpretation—clay tablets stretching back to the early third millennium BCE. For practitioners of medical astrology, these texts matter as origin: the conceptual foundation upon which all subsequent oneiromantic traditions were built, whether by elaboration or reaction. Here, in the river valleys between the Tigris and the Euphrates, astrology and oneiromancy were born as twin sciences. The conviction that stars and dreams speak the same divine language first received systematic articulation.

The Mesopotamian dream stands at the external pole of a spectrum running through Egyptian threshold-crossing to Chinese internal diagnosis. In this earliest literate tradition, the dream is visitation—a deity or spirit entering the sleeping chamber, standing at the dreamer's head, delivering a message from the divine council. The sleeper is a witness, not an author. The dream arrives from outside, carrying information about external reality: the will of the gods, the fate of kingdoms, the prognosis of illness.

The same gods who inscribed fate in planetary movements inscribed it in nocturnal visions. Both media required trained interpreters; both yielded actionable intelligence about the future; both belonged to a unified science of reading divine intention from observable signs. The scribal academies that produced *Enūma Anu Enlil*, the great celestial omen series, also produced *Iškar Zaqīqu*, the dream omen series. The methodologies were identical because the subject matter was identical: heavenly writing, whether traced across the night sky or across the sleeping mind.

## Zaqīqu: The Wind-Spirit and the Dream-God

Mesopotamians conceptualized dream experience through the *zaqīqu*—a term variously translated as "spirit," "phantom," or "wind." The *zaqīqu* was a component of the human person capable of separating from the body during sleep, traveling to other realms, or receiving visitation from external spirits. The name derives from the verb "to blow"—the dream-spirit moves like wind, invisible but powerful, crossing boundaries that constrain the waking body.

This wind-spirit was personified in the deity Zaqīqu, god of dreams, mediator between the divine realm and the human sleeper. When the great gods wished to communicate with mortals, Zaqīqu carried their messages into sleeping minds. The dreamer did not generate content; the dreamer received transmission. The *zaqīqu* within the sleeper served as a receptor—antenna tuned to frequencies inaudible to waking consciousness.

The vulnerability of sleep receives careful attention in Mesopotamian sources. When a person's relationship with their personal protective deity was intact, a spiritual canopy sheltered the sleeping *zaqīqu* from malevolent interference. If the personal god was angered or absent—through transgression or ritual pollution—this protection lifted. The unguarded *zaqīqu* lay open to demonic predation, producing the nightmares and symptomatic dreams that signaled spiritual crisis. Dream quality served as diagnostic indicator: clear, meaningful dreams suggested intact divine protection; confused, terrifying dreams suggested its absence.

Practitioners familiar with Chinese medicine will recognize structural parallels. The *zaqīqu* functions analogously to the *hún* in Chinese cosmology—the ethereal component that wanders during sleep, while the *pò* remains with the body. Egyptian tradition distinguished the *bꜣ* (mobile soul-bird) from aspects that stayed with the corpse. Greek *pneuma* carries the same wind etymology. These convergences suggest historical transmission, independent recognition of something real about human experience during sleep, or both.

# Šiṭir Šamê: Dreams as Heavenly Writing

The conceptual key for medical astrologers lies in the Mesopotamian phrase *šiṭir šamê*—"the writing of heaven." This term applied equally to celestial phenomena and dreams. Both belonged to the same epistemic category: inscriptions made by the gods, legible to those trained in reading divine script. The stars wrote across the night sky; dreams wrote across the sleeping mind. Same authors, same language, different tablets.

The great celestial omen series *Enūma Anu Enlil*—"When Anu and Enlil"—compiled observations of lunar, solar, planetary, stellar, and meteorological phenomena into a comprehensive reference work of some seventy tablets. Its methodology was identical to the Dream Omen series: correlations accumulated through generations of systematic observation. "If the moon at its appearance is surrounded by a halo and Scorpius stands in it: there will be a fire in the land." "If a man dreams of eating a raven, his income will increase." Grammatical structure, epistemological assumptions, and practical applications—all are continuous across celestial and oneiric divination.

This equation grounds all subsequent astrological dream interpretation. When Guido Bonatti, two millennia later, uses the ninth house and its planetary ruler to assess dream veracity, he operates within a framework Mesopotamian scribes would have recognized: celestial configurations and dream content as parallel expressions of divine intention, mutually illuminating, appropriately read together.

## *The Three Paths of the Sky*

Mesopotamian astronomers organized the heavens into three bands, each assigned to a ruling deity. The northern band—stars that never set, circling the pole—belonged to Enlil, king of the gods. The central band, encompassing the celestial equator where sun, moon, and planets traveled, belonged to Anu, god of heaven. The southern band, containing stars that rose and set but spent much of their time below the horizon, belonged to Ea, god of wisdom and the watery abyss.

This tripartite division provided the framework within which all celestial observation occurred. When astrologers assessed timing for dream incubation or evaluated which stellar influences shaped a particular dream, they worked within this cosmological architecture.

The Path of the Moon—the band through which the moon traveled in its monthly circuit—held particular significance for dream work. Eighteen constellations marked this path, corresponding roughly to what later traditions would call the zodiac, though the

Mesopotamian conception preceded and differed from the twelve-sign system that emerged in the late first millennium BCE. The moon's passage through these stations governed ritual timing, including rites intended to induce or interpret dreams.

## *Lunar Timing and Dream Potency*

The lunar cycle structured all Mesopotamian religious and divinatory practices; dream work was no exception. The night is divided into three watches (*maṣṣarāti*): the Watch of the People (evening), the Watch of the Gods (midnight), and the Watch of the Morning (dawn). Dreams in the first watch reflected the day's residue. Dreams in the second watch, when the soul traveled deepest, carried the greatest spiritual significance. Dreams in the third watch were prescriptive, providing specific guidance for action. The monthly lunar phases similarly governed dream potency: the full moon (*Šapattu*) marked the zenith of noetic light, when dreams were most likely true and prognostic; the dark moon (*Bubbulum*) opened communication with the dead. (For detailed lunar timing tables, see Appendix D.)

This attention to celestial timing persists through every subsequent tradition of dream incubation. Greek Asclepian sanctuaries, Egyptian temple sleep, medieval electional astrology applied to dream-seeking—all inherit the Mesopotamian recognition that the sky's configuration affects the quality and significance of dreams received. The practitioner who times incubation to the lunar phase operates within a tradition that Babylonian scribes would have endorsed.

## *Astrology as Authenticator*

The Mesopotamian divinatory hierarchy made the relationship between stars and dreams explicit. Dreams were valid sources of omen but also subjective—vulnerable to distortion by the dreamer's condition, demonic interference, or misremembering. The high sciences of the court—astrology and extispicy (reading entrails)—served to authenticate dream messages.

A king who received an alarming dream did not act immediately; he consulted astrologers and liver-diviners to verify whether celestial and visceral signs confirmed the dream's content. The astrologer examined recent and upcoming celestial phenomena: had there been significant planetary configurations? What omens had the moon displayed? Did current stellar positions support or contradict the dream's apparent message? If stars and liver agreed with the dream, the message was validated. If they contradicted it, the dream might be dismissed as demonic deception or digestive disturbance.

This practice grounds the technique Hellenistic and medieval practitioners would develop: using astrological methods to evaluate dreams. The dream provides initial data; the chart provides verification. Neither source complete without the other. Mesopotamian practice models the integration this volume advocates: celestial and oneiric evidence read as complementary inscriptions of a single divine intention.

## The Iškar Zaqīqu: Structure and Method

The primary textual monument of Mesopotamian dream science is the *Iškar Zaqīqu*—the Series of the Dream-God—an eleven-tablet compendium preserved in the library of the Assyrian king Ashurbanipal at Nineveh (seventh century BCE), compiled from sources reaching back to the Old Babylonian period a thousand years earlier. This Assyrian Dream Book holds the accumulated wisdom of generations of scholar-priests who recorded dreams, tracked outcomes, and organized findings into systematic reference works.

The series stood alongside *Enūma Anu Enlil* (celestial omens) and *Bārûtu* (extispicy) as one of three great divinatory compendia. All three shared methodology, format, and underlying assumptions: the gods communicate through signs; signs can be systematically catalogued; trained interpreters can read what the gods have written. The dream book was court science, produced and maintained by the same scholarly elite who tracked planetary movements and examined sacrificial livers.

*Table 3.1. Mesopotamian Dream Tablet Structure*

| Tablet | Contents | Function |
|---|---|---|
| I | Waking incantations | Secure favorable outcomes; neutralize threatening portents while meaning remains malleable |
| II–IX | Omen manual | Conditional correlations: 'If a man dreams X, then Y will occur' |
| X–XI | *Namburbi* rituals | Avert evil portended by negative dreams; transform diagnosis into intervention |

This tripartite structure—prayer, interpretation, remediation—mirrors *Enūma Anu Enlil* and establishes the template for all subsequent oneiromantic practice.

### *The Phoneme Method*

The logic connecting image to outcome often operated through sound—words that resembled each other phonetically were linked in reality. The gods had structured the cosmos through language. Phonetic resemblance was designed, not an accident. The interpreter who heard the echo accessed encoded meaning.

Three examples: If a man is given *miḫru*-wood, he shall have no rival (*māḫiru*). If a man eats a raven (*āribu*), his income (*irbu*) increases. If a man eats human flesh (*šēru*), great riches (*šarû*) will come. Sound, not symbol. Divine language, not human sentiment.

This interpretive technology deserves more than antiquarian notice. The principle—that meaning travels through phonetic channels the conscious mind does not control—appears in dream interpretation across cultures. The dreaming mind operates closer to divine inscription than waking cognition. It communicates through these channels naturally.

## Namburbi: Ritual Remediation

When a dream portended ill, the Mesopotamians did not accept fate. The *namburbi* rituals—"undoing" or "loosening"—dissolved the connection between omen and outcome. Warning, not fate; ritual response could redirect trajectory. This principle underlies all subsequent traditions of astrological remediation. The *āšipu* (exorcist-priest) conducted these ceremonies in three phases:

> *Preparation* involved separating ritual space, purifying the dreamer through washing, and offering prayers to Šamaš (Sun, justice) or Ea (wisdom, the watery depths). Timing was astronomically determined—certain lunar phases and stellar risings favored loosening.
>
> *Transfer* constituted the central action. The dreamer recounted the threatening dream into a proxy healing object—a lump of clay, a figurine, a portion of bread. Incantations specified that the evil portent should move from the dreamer into the substitute. The dream's negative charge was extracted from the person who received it.
>
> *Dissolution* completed the ritual. The substitute was destroyed—thrown into the river, buried, burned. Salt dissolved; knotted cords untied. The dreamer departed without looking back.

The therapeutic logic endures: diagnosis implies prognosis; prognosis enables intervention. The threatening dream is a warning—an opportunity to act before manifestation. This is the logic of astrological remediation. When a medieval astrologer prescribes a Saturn talisman to mitigate a transit revealed in a dream, the architecture is Mesopotamian. The *namburbi* established that the future, though written by the gods, remains negotiable.

## Gula and the Astral-Somatic Dimension

The goddess Gula governed healing and biliary function. Mesopotamians associated dream quality with digestive health—disturbed liver, disturbed dreams; settled digestion, clear reception. This somatic dimension persists through Greek humoral theory into medieval medicine, where the liver remained central to both health and dream quality.

Gula's celestial home was The Goat (MUL.ÙZ)—Lyra, dominated by Vega. Vega rises in the northeast during late spring and stands overhead on summer nights, when Gula's healing influence is most accessible. Her sacred dog occupied the neighboring constellation, now Hercules. Healer and companion together in the summer heavens.

Temple practices at Gula's sanctuaries included placing patients under the stars overnight. Celestial incubation: the sick person sleeping beneath the goddess's star, receiving both dream guidance and astral therapeutic power. The visible constellation served as a conduit—not symbolic but functionally effective. Priests positioned patients so Vega's light fell upon them, stellar rays carrying Gula's healing into the sleeping body.

Astral irradiation extended beyond incubation. Medications and amulets were "set in the star" (*ina kakkabi tušbāt*)—exposed to stellar influence overnight to absorb celestial power, then administered, carrying stellar virtue into the body. Direct ancestor of charging talismans under planetary hours or stellar risings.

The Gula material establishes persistent principles. Dream clarity correlates with hepatobiliary function. Specific celestial bodies govern specific healing functions; visible presence facilitates transmission. Timing matters: Gula's influence peaks when Vega rides high. Objects can be charged with stellar power—the foundation of all talismanic medicine.

## Royal Dreams: Celestial Legitimation

Dreams legitimated royal power. Gudea of Lagash (circa 2100 BCE) recorded dreams commanding him to rebuild the temple of Ningirsu. A giant figure, "huge as heaven and earth," appeared with Nisaba, patron of writing and astronomy, holding a golden stylus and tablet of stars. The tablet held the temple's blueprint—inscribed in the heavens, to be built on earth.

Nisaba's star-tablet provided the celestial template for terrestrial structure. The temple mirrored cosmic architecture—orientations aligned to cardinal directions, rituals timed to celestial cycles, its existence connecting earth and heaven. The dream revealed not that Gudea should build but how: in accordance with a celestial pattern.

Gudea woke "shaking and trembling" and sought interpretation from Nanše, goddess of dream divination. Astrologers then verified the dream against celestial signs. Only after triangulation—dream confirmed by interpretation and celestial observation—did building commence. The discipline of reading sky and dream together was *de rigueur*.

A millennium later, Ashurbanipal employed the same method. Before the war against Elam, Ishtar of Arbela—Venus—appeared to a seer armed for battle, announcing she would fight for Assyria. Astrologers verified timing: Venus rising as Morning Star, Ishtar in warrior aspect. Dream provided an omen; stars confirmed.

## The Hierarchy of Signs

Different methods held different prestige. Stars could not lie; the liver displayed configurations multiple observers could verify. Dreams were more subjective—passing through the individual's *zaqīqu*, potentially distorted by personal condition, demonic interference, and faulty memory.

The hierarchy was explicit. *Extispicy*—examination of the sacrificial liver—ranked highest for military decisions. Astrology ranked nearly as high, *Enūma Anu Enlil* guiding state policy. Oneiromancy ranked below, providing initial leads that the higher sciences would verify or reject.

Yet the three were complementary. A complete assessment integrated all evidence: dream checked against celestial configurations, confirmed by the liver. Concordance produced confidence; discordance demanded investigation. The principle applies to contemporary practice: dream evaluated against natal chart, horary chart, and active transits. Multiple streams yield more reliable guidance than any single stream.

Using astrological evidence to evaluate dreams—direct precedent for Hellenistic and medieval technique. Bonatti's ninth-house protocols continue this practice. The practitioner who examines Moon's condition, the ninth lord's dignity, and aspects active on the night of a dream operates within a tradition Mesopotamian astrologers would recognize.

## The Night as Revelation

For the Mesopotamians, night was not darkness but disclosure. The same gods who inscribed fate in planetary movements inscribed it in the visions of sleepers. Both were *šiṭir šamê*—heavenly writing, legible to those who learned the script. This conviction that celestial and oneiric phenomena belong to a single system of divine communication established the architecture within which all subsequent traditions would work.

The legacy is substantial. From Mesopotamia: the equation of stellar and dream omens—same format, same empirical accumulation, same confidence that observation yields correlation. Lunar timing for incubation. Stellar irradiation—charging objects with celestial power. The insight is that meaning travels through phonetic channels beneath conscious intention. The *namburbi* principle: ominous dreams can be dissolved; diagnosis implies prognosis; prognosis enables intervention. Triangulation—stars verifying what the night revealed.

Yet something remained unaddressed. In the Mesopotamian model, the dream arrives from outside—deity visits sleeper, message enters mind—and the sleeper's nature scarcely matters. The same dream descending upon two individuals carries the same meaning. The constitution is noise, not a signal. The liver might cloud reception, but interpretation proceeds as though dreamers were interchangeable vessels, differing in clarity of reception, not character of response.

### *The Nile Valley developed a different understanding.*

Egyptian oneiromancy, preserved in the Ramesside Dream Book (Chester Beatty III, circa 1220 BCE), introduces threshold consciousness. The term for dream, *resut*, derives from "to awaken"—not unconsciousness but awakening into a liminal state where communication becomes possible. The dreamer stands at a boundary. What crosses registers differently depending on who stands there.

The Egyptians recognized two constitutional types: followers of Horus and followers of Seth. The same image—face in a mirror, date harvest, appearance of an animal—portended differently for each. The Mesopotamian interpretation moved directly from image to outcome. Egyptian interpretation introduced a mediating variable: if X, then Y for this type, but Z for that type. The message remained external but passed through a constitutional filter.

Crucial movement along the spectrum from external to internal. The source remains outside—gods, spirits, forces governing fate. But now registration depends on the inherent nature. Same transmission, different instruments, different readings.

Egypt also localized dreams in the body. The Four Sons of Horus assigned organ governance—lungs, stomach, intestines, liver—anticipating Chinese organ-spirit correlations. The divine message still arrives from outside, but the body that receives it now matters.

The next chapter traces Egyptian development. From Mesopotamia to the Nile. From dreams arriving uniformly to dreams registering constitutionally. From interchangeable vessels to embodied types. The threshold opens.

## Sources

Butler, S.A.L. *Mesopotamian Conceptions of Dreams and Dream Rituals.* Münster: Ugarit-Verlag, 1998.

Hunger, Hermann, and David Pingree. *Astral Sciences in Mesopotamia.* Leiden: Brill, 1999.

Noegel, Scott B. *Nocturnal Ciphers: The Allusive Language of Dreams in the Ancient Near East.* New Haven: American Oriental Society, 2007.

Oppenheim, A. Leo. *The Interpretation of Dreams in the Ancient Near East, with a Translation of an Assyrian Dream-Book.* Transactions of the American Philosophical Society 46.3. Philadelphia: American Philosophical Society, 1956.

Reiner, Erica. *Astral Magic in Babylonia.* Transactions of the American Philosophical Society 85.4. Philadelphia: American Philosophical Society, 1995.

Rochberg, Francesca. *The Heavenly Writing: Divination, Horoscopy, and Astronomy in Mesopotamian Culture*. Cambridge: Cambridge University Press, 2004.

Zgoll, Annette. *Traum und Welterleben im antiken Mesopotamien*. Münster: Ugarit-Verlag, 2006.

# Chapter Four

# The Egyptian Threshold

*wḥ' ts.t n.t rsw.t*

*"To untie the knot of the dream."*

—Papyrus Chester Beatty III

On the external-internal spectrum, Egypt stands at the threshold. The dream still arrives from outside—gods and spirits communicate through sleep—but who receives the message shapes what it means. The Horian and Sethian constitutions filter the same divine communication differently. External message meets embodied reception. This is the first movement toward internalization.

## The Dream as Awakening

The Egyptian word for dream tells us something essential. *Resut* (*rsw.t*) derives from the verb meaning "to awake" or "to be watchful." The dream is not unconsciousness but heightened vigilance—an awakening into perception unavailable to ordinary sight.

Scribes reinforced this through hieroglyphics. *Resut* was written with the open eye determinative—dreamer aligned with seeing. The dreamer perceives; the dreamer watches. What the dreamer watches is external reality, not internal fantasy—a threshold space where the living encounter gods, blessed dead, supernatural forces otherwise inaccessible.

Egyptian grammar confirms this. One does not 'dream' content into being. One sees a dream. The sleeper is the recipient, not the author. Clinical significance: the dreamer receives communications from forces external to ordinary consciousness—beneficent or malevolent. Received content requires professional interpretation.

Both traditions understood dreams as external communications. But Egypt introduced something new: the dreamer's constitution affects how communications register. The same divine message, passing through different types, produces different meanings. The threshold is not neutral ground.

## Two Natures: Followers of Horus and Seth

The Ramesside Dream Book—the oldest systematic dream interpretation manual in existence, dating to approximately 1220 BCE—divides humanity into two constitutional types: Followers of Horus and Followers of Seth. This division mirrors Egyptian cosmology. The struggle between Horus and Seth—order against chaos, fertile valley against barren desert—manifests not only among the gods but within individual human beings.

The mantic value of any dream depends on which type the dreamer embodies. A single symbol carries opposite meaning depending on the dreamer's inherent nature.

## *The Horus-like or Horian Constitution*

The Follower of Horus aligns with Maat—cosmic order, truth, justice, proper function. The sources characterize Horian individuals by the "Open Eye": falcon-like vigilance, clarity, and measured awareness. Horian behavior tends toward stability, adherence to tradition, and appropriate social conduct.

Celestially, the Horian type corresponds to the circumpolar stars—the *ikhemu-sek*, the "Imperishable" that never sets below the horizon, eternally visible, eternally ordered. These stars provided the template for immortality. The pyramid shafts were aligned to them so the pharaoh's soul could join their eternal circuit.

When Horians fall ill, their disturbances typically involve internal depletion—the "skipping" of the heart, weakness at the vital center. Treatment requires restoration rather than defense.

## *The Sethian Constitution*

The Follower of Seth aligns with Isfet—chaos, disruption, the forces opposing order. Physical markers identify the type: red hair, curly hair, freckles, ruddy complexion. Red was Seth's color, written in the ink that designated danger.

Beyond appearance, Sethians manifest characteristic patterns: quarrelsome disposition, proneness to anger, what the sources call "earthy" manners. They gravitate toward intensity, disruption, boundary-crossing. Not moral failings—constitutional tendencies. Alignment with the chaos-power Seth embodies.

Celestially, the Sethian corresponds to Meskhetyu—the Big Dipper, depicted in Egyptian star maps as the Foreleg of the Bull, shown bound by chains and guarded by a hippopotamus goddess to prevent Seth from causing chaos in the heavens. Even the stars must be restrained.

Sethians are particularly vulnerable to nightmares—*dw rsw.t*, "bad dreams"—involving assault by hostile dead or demonic entities. Constitutional alignment with chaos renders them open to chaotic attack. But they possess native capacity to function within chaotic conditions that would overwhelm the Horian.

## *Interpretive Adjustment*

The practitioner establishes the constitutional type before interpreting dream content. Physical markers provide an initial indication; behavioral history and dream disturbance pattern confirm the assessment.

For Horians, standard interpretations apply. For Sethians, systematic adjustment. A dream of fire—portending destruction of domestic order for the Horian—may indicate a favorable return to primordial power for the Sethian. Same image, different constitutions, opposite meanings.

Here, Egypt advances beyond Mesopotamia. Both traditions understood dreams as external communications. Mesopotamia moved directly from image to outcome: if X, then Y. Egypt introduced the receiver as a variable: if X, then Y for this type, but Z for that type. The threshold is not neutral. Who stands there shapes what crosses.

## *Untying the Knot*

The Egyptian term for dream interpretation was *wḥʿ ts.t*—"to untie the knot." The metaphor pervades Egyptian magical literature. Knots bind; knots constrain; knots hold power in fixed form. The dream arrives as bound, meaning—encrypted communication from the divine realm. The interpreter (*wḥʿ-ts.t*, "knot-untier") releases this meaning into comprehensible form.

The method operates through a specific understanding: language participates in reality rather than merely describing it. Words are not arbitrary signs but carriers of essence. The sound of a thing connects to the nature of the thing. This understanding generates the interpretive techniques.

### *Phonetic Resonance*

Mesopotamia discovered the phoneme method—meaning encoded in sound. Egypt formalized it as paronomasia, interpretive punning. Not frivolous wordplay. Phonetic resemblance reveals a real connection. Same sound, linked referents.

Dreaming of white bread (*ḥḏ*) portends the face "lighting up" (*ḥḏ*) with joy—same root, substance to outcome. Dreaming of donkey flesh (*ꜥꜣ*) portends greatness (*ꜥꜣ*)—same consonant, same link. The interpreter searches for homophones, near-homophones, and alliterative correspondences bridging image to consequence.

Artemidorus transmitted the method to Rome. When a medieval interpreter finds significance in dream-word sounds, the lineage runs from Babylon to Alexandria to the Latin West.

### *Paradoxical Inversion*

The dream realm operates by laws contrary to waking expectation. Positive valence portends a negative outcome; disturbing images herald a benefit. The threshold inverts.

Copulating with a woman—pleasurable waking—portends mourning. Burying an old man—sorrowful waking—portends flourishing. The interpreter applies systematic inversion where emotional charge runs strong. What appears as joy in the liminal realm manifests as grief; what appears as death manifests as vitality.

## The Ramesside Catalogue

The Dream Book preserved in Papyrus Chester Beatty III provides over two hundred interpretations organized by image. The manuscript's visual organization reinforced interpretation: the word 'BAD' was written in red ink—Seth's color—while all other text appeared in black. Rapid consultation during professional practice required immediate visual discrimination.

Selected entries illustrate the method:

*Table 4.1. Selected Entries from the Ramesside Dream Book*

| Dream Image | Value | Outcome | Mechanism |
|---|---|---|---|
| White bread given | GOOD | Face lights up with joy | Homonymy: ḥḏ (white/bright) |
| Burying an old man | GOOD | Flourishing | Paradoxical inversion |
| Submerging in river | GOOD | Purification from evils | Ritual association |
| Eating crocodile meat | GOOD | Acting as official | Consuming Sobek's power |
| Penis becoming erect | BAD | Victory for enemies | Antanaclasis: nḫt (stiffening/victory) |
| Face in mirror | BAD | Another wife (rival) | Reflection = duplication |
| Copulating with woman | BAD | Mourning | Paradoxical inversion |
| Teeth falling out | BAD | Dependents will die | Phonetic: ḥry (below/dependents) |
| Bed catching fire | BAD | Driving away wife | Destruction of domestic center |

# The Four Sons of Horus: Dreams and the Organs

Egyptian mummification removed four organs for separate preservation: lungs, stomach, intestines, and liver. Each was placed in a canopic jar guarded by one of the Four Sons of Horus—protective deities maintaining integrity through eternity. Hapy, baboon-headed, guarded the lungs; Duamutef, jackal-headed, the stomach; Qebehsenuef, falcon-headed, the intestines; Imsety, human-headed, the liver.

Their governance extended beyond death. During embodied life, these deities regulated the corresponding organs and communicated through dreams.

Later dream books—Demotic texts from the Ptolemaic period—preserve a system correlating dream animals with these deities. The mechanism is feeding. Feed an animal in the dream, establish a relationship with the deity manifest in that form. Feed a baboon, engage Hapy—power localizes in the lungs. Feed a jackal, engage Duamutef—power settles in the stomach.

The system extends beyond the Four Sons. Feed an ibis, enter a relationship with Thoth, lord of wisdom, whose seat is the heart. Each deity-animal pairing maps to specific anatomy. The dream becomes diagnostic: which organ calls for attention, which deity requires propitiation.

### *Clinical Application*

When a patient reports feeding an animal in a dream, the practitioner identifies the deity-organ relationship and examines that system. The dream may precede symptomatic manifestation—the deity draws attention to their protected organ before physical symptoms emerge.

Feeding the baboon warrants assessment of respiratory function. Feeding the jackal indicates stomach and digestion. Feeding the falcon points to intestinal health. Feeding a human figure concerns the liver. Feeding the bull—most significant—indicates the heart requires attention, seat of consciousness and blood-governance.

Genuine diagnostic technology. The dream provides prodromal indication; the practitioner investigates before symptoms fully manifest. Egypt developed organ-specific dream diagnosis two thousand years before Classical Chinese Medicine elaborated its own system of organ-spirit correlations.

## The Binary Oracle: Signs of Maat and Isfet

For simple yes/no questions, Egyptian practice employed a binary oracle. The practitioner posed a question before incubation and requested a sign: affirmative or negative, proceed or desist.

Yes: plant life and water. The signature of Maat—divine blessing, conditions favorable to flourishing. Water and vegetation represent the Nile's gift, the annual inundation renewing Egypt's fertility. This sign indicates the proposed action aligns with cosmic order.

No: fire and iron. The signature of Isfet—divine obstruction, conditions hostile to the endeavor. Fire consumes; iron cuts and wounds. Seth's signatures—desert heat, foreign weapon, forces opposing Egyptian order. This sign indicates the proposed action opposes divine will.

Constitutional type modifies interpretation. For the Horian, fire/iron indicates a clear prohibition—ordered nature cannot thrive under a chaotic signature. For the Sethian, the same sign may indicate temporary hindrance rather than absolute prohibition. The Sethian has a native capacity to function within chaos.

# Temple Sleep

Deliberate induction of oracular dreams—temple incubation—followed careful ritual preparation. The practitioner did not simply sleep and hope for meaning. Specific conditions ensured divine communication could occur.

## *Preparation*

Three days of fasting and sexual abstinence preceded the incubation night. Withdrawal from ordinary appetites prepared for extraordinary encounter.

The sleep space was cleansed with aromatic smoke. The sleeper rested on white sheets, purity required for a divine approach. Constitutional type determined dietary modification: Sethians required cooling foods—lettuce, cucumber—to prevent internal heat flaring during ritual sleep. Horians avoided cold substances that would weaken the heart-center.

## *The Akephalos*

A drawing of the Akephalos—the "Headless One," a form of Osiris as impartial judge—was placed under the pillow. Surrounded by magical formulae, this figure functioned as an intermediary, compelling an honest divine response.

The Akephalos is neither beneficent nor maleficent. Without head—without the ordinary seat of will and intention—he represents impartiality beyond personal interest. His function: compel the invoked deity to speak truth without evasion. The sleeper places their question under the protection of this neutral arbiter.

### *Memory and Protection*

Divine communication received during sleep requires retention upon waking. Practitioners applied preparations to the lips before sleep: honey mixed with mugwort (*Artemisia vulgaris*) and powdered magnetite. Honey served as a carrier; mugwort enhanced dream vividness; magnetite attracted divine communication and fixed it in memory.

Ritual sleep required protection. Images of Bes, the protective dwarf-deity, and Taweret, the hippopotamus goddess, were placed on the headrest to ward off nightmare intrusion. Sethians required particular attention, given their constitutional vulnerability to demonic assault.

Upon waking, the dreamer immediately recorded or reported the dream before any other activity. The liminal state between sleep and full waking preserved access; delay risked losing crucial details.

## What Egypt Teaches

The Egyptian system advances oneiromantic practice in ways that persist through all subsequent traditions.

*Constitutional mediation.* The same dream means different things for different people. This recognition—obvious once stated, revolutionary in practice—transforms interpretation from mechanical correlation to individualized assessment. The practitioner must know who the dreamer is before interpreting what they dreamed.

*Organ-dream correlation.* Dreams indicate developing pathology before symptoms manifest. The Four Sons of Horus system reads dream animals as prodromal indicators pointing to specific organ systems. This diagnostic technology anticipates later developments in Classical Chinese and Greek medicine.

*The threshold principle.* The dream is not mere unconsciousness but awakening into a liminal space where different laws apply. Paradoxical inversion, phonetic resonance, symbolic condensation—not interpretive impositions but recognitions of how the threshold realm operates.

*Prepared incubation.* Meaningful dreams can be sought, not merely received. The seeking requires preparation—physical, psychological, and ritual. The practitioner who understands incubation protocol can guide patients toward dreams that provide diagnostic or therapeutic information.

*Binary clarity.* Sometimes the question is simple: yes or no, proceed or desist. The plant/water versus fire/iron system provides a framework for receiving and interpreting direct divine guidance on specific inquiries.

## Toward the East

Egypt refined what Mesopotamia established. The external message remains external—gods and spirits communicate through dreams—but the dreamer's constitution shapes how that message registers. The threshold is not neutral glass but a colored lens. Different constitutions filter the same light differently.

Traditions east of Egypt pushed further toward internalization. Indian dream theory, rooted in the *svapna* teachings of the Upanishads, locates dream experience within the subtle body and correlates it with the play of the three *guṇas*—the fundamental qualities constituting all manifest reality. The dreamer becomes not merely a recipient but a participant; the dream itself becomes a state of consciousness with its own ontological status.

Classical Chinese Medicine completed the internalization. Dreams emerge from organ-spirit dynamics within the body itself. The *hún* wanders during sleep not to receive external messages but because its relationship with blood and Liver requires this nocturnal activity. What appears in the dream indicates the state of internal organs, the balance of *qì*, the condition of the Five Spirits. The external has become fully internal.

But Egypt stands at the threshold—appropriately, given its organizing metaphor. Neither fully external like Mesopotamia nor fully internal like China, the Egyptian system recognizes that communication requires both sender and receiver, and that who receives shapes what is received. This insight persists through all subsequent developments. The natal chart modifying dream interpretation in later astrological practice descends from Egyptian constitutional typology: the same celestial message, filtered through different births, produces different meanings.

The chapter that follows traces Indian development, where the dream becomes a distinct state of consciousness and the subtle body provides the anatomy of nocturnal experience.

*Note: For detailed treatment of the Egyptian decanal system, the twelve hours of the underworld, and planetary personifications, see Appendix B: Egyptian Astronomical Framework.*

## Sources

Betz, Hans Dieter, ed. *The Greek Magical Papyri in Translation, Including the Demotic Spells*. 2nd ed. Chicago: University of Chicago Press, 1992.

Gardiner, Alan H. *Hieratic Papyri in the British Museum, Third Series: Chester Beatty Gift*. 2 vols. London: British Museum, 1935.

Noegel, Scott B. 'On Puns and Divination: Egyptian Dream Exegesis from a Comparative Perspective.' In *Ancient Divination and Experience*, edited by Lindsay G. Driediger-Murphy and Esther Eidinow, 95–119. Oxford: Oxford University Press, 2019.

Quack, Joachim Friedrich. 'Word Play in the Ramesside Dream Manual.' In *Puns and Pundits: Word Play in the Hebrew Bible and Ancient Near Eastern Literature*, edited by Scott B. Noegel, 193–212. Bethesda: CDL Press, 2000.

Ritner, Robert K. *The Mechanics of Ancient Egyptian Magical Practice*. Studies in Ancient Oriental Civilization 54. Chicago: Oriental Institute, 1993.

Szpakowska, Kasia. *Behind Closed Eyes: Dreams and Nightmares in Ancient Egypt*. Swansea: Classical Press of Wales, 2003.

Szpakowska, Kasia, ed. *Through a Glass Darkly: Magic, Dreams, and Prophecy in Ancient Egypt*. Swansea: Classical Press of Wales, 2006.

Volten, Aksel. *Demotische Traumdeutung (Pap. Carlsberg XIII und XIV verso)*. Analecta Aegyptiaca 3. Copenhagen: Munksgaard, 1942.

## Chapter Five

# The Vedic Framework

स्वप्नो हि देवानां दूतः

*svapno hi devānāṃ dūtaḥ*

*"The dream is the messenger of the gods."*

—Bṛhat Saṃhitā 68.3

The Vedic tradition stands midway on the external-internal spectrum. The dream remains messenger—*dūta*—carrying communication from beyond the dreamer. Yet Indian frameworks acknowledge that humoral imbalance and mental states can generate imagery indistinguishable from prophetic content. The tradition preserves divine sourcing while making room for bodily causation. What India contributes is precision: validation protocols distinguishing genuine transmission from somatic noise, timing frameworks predicting manifestation, and remedial technology redirecting unfavorable portents.

## The Dream as Messenger

The Sanskrit *svapna* encompasses both dream state and dream content—the mode of consciousness and its productions cannot be separated. This linguistic fact points to something the Vedic tradition understood: the dream is not a thing that happens to consciousness, but a form consciousness takes. To dream is to enter a distinct mode of knowing.

Varāhamihira's sixth-century *Bṛhat Saṃhitā* opens its dream chapter with a declaration: the dream is the messenger of the gods. Not metaphor. Not psychological projection. Messenger—*dūta*—one who carries communication from elsewhere. The dream arrives bearing news. The interpreter's task is to read the message accurately and respond appropriately.

This chapter presents the Vedic framework as it integrates with Jyotiṣa. The system offers sophisticated tools: validation protocols distinguishing prophetic dreams from mental noise, timing frameworks predicting when dreams will manifest, planetary signatures identifying which celestial influence predominates, and remedial measures redirecting unfavorable portents. Where Egypt introduced constitutional mediation—the same dream meaning different things for different types—India introduces temporal precision and remedial technology.

# The Vessel of Sleep

Before a dream can speak, sleep must receive the dreamer. Sleep quality determines dream quality—coherence, depth, capacity to carry meaning. In Vedic astrology, this receptive vessel is governed by the twelfth house, *Vyaya Bhāva*—the House of Loss.

The name points to what must be surrendered for sleep to occur: the grip of waking consciousness, the vigilance of senses, the assertion of ego. Only through this loss does the dreamer gain access to the imaginal realm. The twelfth house is the terminal point of the zodiacal circuit—repository for all that must be dissolved or transcended. It governs consciousness in the absence of external sensory input.

Three planets govern sleep physiology. Mercury rules the nervous system—the switching mechanism that allows the mind to release the day. When Mercury is afflicted in the twelfth, the switch fails; the mind continues its daytime loop, sleep fragments, and depth never arrives. Moon governs the emotional body and its tidal rhythms; lunar affliction produces restless sleep as unprocessed feeling surfaces in nightmare form. Jupiter expands whatever it touches; well-placed in the twelfth, Jupiter deepens sleep and opens the dream channel to prophetic material.

Each planet colors the twelfth house distinctly when placed there. Sun diminishes vitality during sleep—natives rise tired despite adequate hours. Mars brings heat and agitation; these natives toss, grind teeth, and wake with muscular tension. Saturn delays sleep onset and may produce heavy, dreamless periods followed by disturbing imagery. Rāhu intensifies the dream state to the point of confusion; the native may struggle to distinguish dream from waking, or experience vivid nightmares. Sleep paralysis correlates strongly with Rāhu's presence here.

Ketu, the south lunar node and *Mokṣa Kāraka* (Significator of Liberation), thins the veil between worlds. These natives often report astral travel, lucid dreaming, or encounters with deceased relatives. The boundary that ordinarily separates sleeping from waking consciousness becomes permeable.

# Validating Prophetic Dreams

Not every dream carries prophetic weight. The Vedic tradition developed rigorous criteria for distinguishing genuine communication from mental processing. Before interpreting dream content, the practitioner must establish whether the dream warrants interpretation at all.

## *The Luminary Connection*

Classical texts ground validation in the luminaries. Sleeping represents darkness—a kind of death in which external awareness ceases. Dreams emerge only when light penetrates this darkness. That light can come only from the Sun and Moon, since other planets possess no inherent luminosity.

Validation requires casting a chart for the approximate time of dreaming. The Ascendant must show a demonstrable connection to the Sun or Moon for a dream to carry predictive significance. The *Bṛhat Saṃhitā* specifies: Sun occupying the Ascendant; Moon aspecting the Ascendant; Leo (the Sun's sign) on the Descendant; or Sun in the Ascendant aspected by Moon. The connection must appear either in the *Rāśī* (sign chart) or the *Navāṃśa* (ninth divisional chart).

Without a luminary connection, the experience may constitute mental wandering rather than prophetic communication. The circuit lacks light; the message lacks authority.

## *The Broken Dream*

A crucial principle concerns the dreamer's behavior upon waking. The *Praśna Mārga* states that if the dreamer wakes from the dream and then returns to sleep, the dream loses its prophetic charge—it 'has got no signification.' The person must either wake to the day directly or not wake at all after the dream.

The logic is electrical: the prophetic charge dissipates when consciousness interrupts, then resumes the sleep cycle. The circuit breaks; the message fails to ground itself in waking awareness. Dreams that wake the dreamer and keep them awake carry weight. Dreams from which the dreamer drifts back to sleep do not.

# Seven Types of Dreams

The *Suśruta Saṃhitā* provides a sevenfold classification clarifying which dreams warrant interpretation. Only one category—the sixth—requires timing analysis and carries prophetic significance.

*Table 5.1. Seven Types of Dreams (Suśruta Saṃhitā)*

| Type | Sanskrit | Source / Nature |
|---|---|---|
| 1 | Dṛṣṭa | Seen during the day (day residue) |
| 2 | Śruta | Heard about from others |
| 3 | Anubhūta | Previously experienced |
| 4 | Prārthita | Desired or wished for |
| 5 | Kalpita | Imagined or fantasized |
| 6 | Bhāvika | Prophetic (timing rules apply) |
| 7 | Doṣaja | Caused by humoral imbalance |

The first five categories reflect psychological processing: day residue, memory, wish fulfillment, and fantasy. The seventh reflects pathology: dreaming of fire when *Pitta* runs high, of water when *Kapha* dominates, of flying or falling when *Vāta* is disturbed.

Only *Bhāvika* dreams carry prophetic weight. Only these require timing analysis. The practitioner's first task is classification: does this dream belong to category six, or does it reflect one of the other six sources?

From the clinical perspective, a *Doṣaja* dream serves diagnosis—it reveals the patient's current humoral state. A *Bhāvika* dream serves as a prognosis—it reveals the trajectory.

# The Four Watches

Vedic tradition divides the night into four watches (*yāma* or *prahara*), assigning different manifestation ranges to dreams occurring in each period. The underlying principle: as night progresses toward dawn, *sattva guṇa* (the quality of purity and clarity) increases. Dreams reflect reality more accurately. The closer a dream to sunrise, the faster it manifests.

*Table 5.2. The Four Watches and Manifestation Timing*

| Watch | Time (Approx.) | Manifestation Range |
|---|---|---|
| First (prathama yāma) | Sunset – 10 PM | Within one year |
| Second (dvitīya yāma) | 10 PM – Midnight | Six to eight months |
| Third (tṛtīya yāma) | Midnight – 3 AM | One to three months |
| Fourth (caturtha yāma) | 3 AM – Sunrise | Ten days to immediate |

Varāhamihira states: 'The effects of dreams seen in the four watches of the night will come to pass within a year, in six or eight months, in three months, and one month or ten days respectively. If seen just before waking up, it will bear fruit almost immediately.'

The *Suśruta Saṃhitā* adds Āyurvedic logic. The first watch falls in the *Kapha* period—mind is clouded, dreams unreliable. The second watch, *Pitta* period—metabolic noise interferes. The third and fourth watches, *Vāta* period—channels clear, mind light, optimal conditions for receiving prophetic transmission.

A dream in the fourth watch, if the dreamer does not sleep again, will surely come true. The Achuar *hora de wayusa* at 3–4 AM, discussed in Chapter Two, corresponds precisely to this window.

# Planetary Signatures in Dreams

The nine planets (*Navagraha*) each govern specific dream content. Recognizing planetary signatures allows the interpreter to identify which celestial influence predominates and correlate dream content with the dreamer's natal chart and current planetary periods.

## *The Luminaries*

Sun (*Sūrya*) governs dreams of blazing fire, red clothes, royalty, temples, father figures, gold, and governmental authority. Solar dreams feature bright light, high places, and figures of dignity.

Moon (*Candra*) governs dreams of women, white flowers, water, gems, jewelry, and emotional encounters. Lunar dreams carry strong feeling-tones and often feature fluid, shifting imagery.

## *The Inner Planets*

Mercury (*Budha*) produces dreams of floating in the air, ascending to heaven, snakes, and news of meritorious acts. The floating quality proves diagnostic—repeated dreams of rising and drifting indicate Mercury's signature.

Venus (*Śukra*) governs dreams of water, swimming, crossing streams, divine blessings, and sexual union.

Mars (*Maṅgala*) governs dreams of gold, coral, bleeding, flesh soaked in blood, fire, conflict, weapons, and surgery.

## *The Outer Planets*

Jupiter (*Guru*) governs dreams of family, sight of gods, association with ascetics, religious ceremonies, children, expansion—generous, optimistic dreams suggesting blessing.

Saturn (*Śani*) governs dreams of climbing mountains, administrative power, journeys through forests, darkness, old age, death, restriction—heavy, serious dreams addressing duty and karmic debt.

## *The Lunar Nodes*

Rāhu (north node) produces dreams of foreigners, deception, smoke, taboo situations, journeys over mountains—the strange, the disorienting, the boundary-violating.

Ketu (south node) produces dreams of spirits, liberation, mysterious events, and past-life material. The *Jātaka Pārijāta* notes that Ketu specifically rules scorpions and venomous creatures; dreams of scorpion attacks point to Ketu's influence.

# The Lunar Mansions

The *nakṣatras* (lunar mansions) are cut finer than the twelve signs. Moon rules *manas* (mind); dreams belong to the Moon. The mansion Moon occupies at dream time sets the tone—each of the twenty-seven spans 13°20′ and carries its own imagery, deity, and psychological quality.

Three temperamental groups organize the mansions:

**Divine (Deva)**: Aśvinī, Mṛgaśirā, Punarvasū, Puṣya, Hasta, Svātī, Anurādhā, Śravaṇa, Revatī. Dreams under these mansions tend toward benevolence, spiritual guidance, auspicious communication.

**Human (Manuṣya)**: Bharaṇī, Rohiṇī, Ārdrā, Pūrva Phalgunī, Uttara Phalgunī, Pūrvāṣāḍhā, Uttarāṣāḍhā, Pūrva Bhādrapadā, Uttara Bhādrapadā. Dreams address worldly matters—family, work, ordinary concerns.

**Demonic (Rākṣasa)**: Kṛttikā, Āśleṣā, Maghā, Citrā, Viśākhā, Jyeṣṭhā, Mūla, Dhaniṣṭhā, Śatabhiṣaj. Dreams involve conflict, ancestral demands, karmic weight, intensity.

Specific signatures emerge from individual mansions. Āśleṣā (Serpent) rules snake dreams and hidden knowledge. Mūla (Root) governs excavation, buried things, and ancestral realms. Maghā (Great) brings ancestors, thrones, and inherited authority. When the Moon's mansion at dream time matches the natal Moon's mansion (*janma nakṣatra*), significance deepens—destiny speaks through the dream.

# The Ninth House Principle

A central principle: dream content and dream results are distinct. The Ascendant of the dream chart reveals what the person dreamed about. But the results—what will actually manifest—are read from the ninth house.

The ninth house represents *bhāgya* (fortune)—fate resulting from merit or demerit in former existences. Dreams fundamentally concern destiny. The *Praśna Mārga* establishes that when crucial events approach, the ninth lord activates dream communication, 'helping you, warning you about it, or telling you about it.'

To read results, the interpreter pivots: the ninth house of the dream chart becomes the new Ascendant—the Dream Ascendant—and all house significations rotate accordingly. What was the tenth house becomes the second from the Dream Ascendant; what was the eleventh becomes the third; and so on. Results are calculated from this rotated framework.

This technique parallels Bonatti's distinction between the ninth house (the dream itself) and other houses (the matters the dream addresses). The traditions converge on the same recognition: dreams speak about destiny, and the ninth house is destiny's house.

## The Method in Practice

A worked example clarifies the ninth-house pivot.

**Dream:** Seeing a white cow in a green field. **Time:** 5:00 AM. **Chart:** Taurus rising, Moon in the ninth house in Capricorn, Venus (Ascendant lord) in the second house.

**Validation:** Moon aspects the Ascendant from the ninth—luminary connection established. Fourth watch timing indicates manifestation within ten days. Taurus rising with white cow imagery confirms earth-sign dream quality.

**Pivot to the ninth:** Capricorn becomes the Dream Ascendant. Saturn (now Ascendant lord) rules practical matters; Moon present indicates emotional significance. The second house from the Dream Ascendant (Aquarius) contains no planets—gains come through steady effort rather than windfall.

**Reading:** Modest material benefit arriving within ten days, likely involving property or food (earth imagery).

A more complex example:

**Dream:** Receiving money from an unknown benefactor. **Time:** 4:30 AM. **Chart:** Sagittarius rising, Jupiter in the second house. The ninth house (Leo) stands empty; Sun as ninth lord occupies the eleventh in Libra, aspected by Jupiter.

**First pass:** Sagittarius Ascendant validates (Jupiter rules); Jupiter in the second points to wealth. But the Ascendant shows what was dreamed, not what manifests.

**Pivot to the ninth:** Leo becomes the Dream Ascendant. Count houses from Leo: Virgo (second) governs gains from the prophecy; Gemini (eleventh) governs hopes fulfilled. Sun, now Ascendant lord, sits third from Leo—courage, initiative, siblings. Jupiter aspects from the sixth—service, daily effort.

**Reading:** Money comes through effort in service, requiring initiative. A sibling or neighbor may figure in. The 'unknown benefactor' dissolves—the dreamer's own work generates the wealth. Fourth watch: expect manifestation within ten days.

## The Āruḍha Lagna: Image and Projection

The *āruḍha lagna* ('Image Ascendant') governs Vedic dream interpretation. The term derives from the Sanskrit root *ā-ruh* (to mount, ascend, climb upon) and signifies that which is mounted or projected—an image, reflection, manifest appearance.

While the Ascendant proper represents the true self, the *āruḍha lagna* represents how that self appears to the world. Dreams operate in the realm of images and projections; the *āruḍha lagna,* therefore, indicates the characteristic imagery, setting, and phenomenal quality of the dream experience itself.

Calculation: Identify the lord of the Ascendant. Count the signs from the Ascendant to that lord's position. Count the same number forward from the lord. The result is the *āruḍha lagna*. (Exception: if the result falls in the first or seventh house from the original, move to the tenth sign instead.)

The sign on the *āruḍha lagna* colors dream imagery. Aries brings temples, towers, and sacred architecture. Taurus brings images of gods, holy statuary, and places where cows are kept. Cancer brings crops, water fields, and agricultural settings. Leo brings hunters and wild creatures. Libra brings merchants, marketplace, and royal themes. Scorpio brings bees, wasps, and poisonous things. Pisces brings the ocean, bathing, gold, and hidden treasures.

## The Construction Chart

Beyond the timed dream chart, practitioners have developed the Construction Chart technique for analyzing complex dreams. This method involves manually placing planets in houses based on the dream's narrative content—a symbolic horoscope capturing the dream's internal logic.

The technique works because the horoscopic framework is a universal grammar of meaning. The twelve houses map all possible domains of human experience; the planets signify all possible agents and forces. Any narrative—waking or dreaming—can be translated into this symbolic language.

The method reverses the usual procedure: instead of deriving meaning from planetary positions determined by astronomical calculation, the interpreter assigns positions based on narrative content and reads the resulting configuration.

### *How It Works*

Identify each significant element in the dream—person, action, object. Assign the appropriate planetary *kāraka* (significator). Place that planet in the house corresponding to the activity.

Example: A dream involving one's mother giving food. Mother = Moon (natural significator). Food and giving = second house (nourishment, sustenance). Construction: Moon is placed in the second house. Inference: nurturing support coming, likely involving actual food or financial help from a maternal figure.

Critical principle: isolate individual activities. One cannot place all dream elements in a single chart. Each activity generates a separate small chart from which specific inferences emerge.

### *Applications*

The *relationship chart* places two significators to examine their house relationship. If the dreamer appears in the seventh house (others, opponents) and an enemy in the first house (self, dominance), the enemy controls the interaction.

The *remedial chart* reverses the process. If a constructed configuration proves inauspicious—Moon (mother) in the sixth house (illness, enemies)—the interpreter asks: what placement would improve the outcome? Moon in the second (nourishment), fourth (home, comfort), or eleventh (gains fulfilled) suggests the direction. The practitioner then translates the favorable configuration into concrete action: offerings to the lunar deity, care directed toward the mother.

This shares the logic of talismanic practice. The chart is not discovered but made, and the making itself constitutes a meaningful act. The dream revealed a pattern; the reconstructed chart reshapes it.

## Recurring Dreams

Recurring dreams require a different approach than single prophetic dreams. Rather than casting a chart for the dream time, the interpreter examines the natal chart for the planetary signature appearing in the dream content, then traces its implications through life unfoldment.

The *Jātaka Pārijāta* guides this method. Recurring dreams of floating point to Mercury's signature. If Mercury occupies severe debility while simultaneously holding dignity by another measure, the tension explains the dream's persistence. Someone with Mercury in Pisces (its fall) but also angular might dream repeatedly of floating or speaking without being heard. The planet is simultaneously weakened and emphasized. The dreams persist until life circumstances address the tension.

The ninth house connection remains relevant. The planet identified in dream imagery typically associates with the ninth lord or occupies the ninth house natally. A troubled Mercury that rules or occupies the ninth has access to the dream channel and will use it.

## Dreams of the Deceased

Dreams featuring deceased relatives hold special significance. The dead may appear to communicate needs—requiring *śrāddha* offerings or other ritual attention—to offer guidance, or to reveal family karmic patterns.

Such dreams are not dismissed as memory or wish-fulfillment but treated as genuine communications requiring an appropriate response. When a deceased relative appears troubled or requests something specific, the traditional response involves ritual feeding of ancestors, charitable giving in the deceased's name, or consultation with a priest regarding appropriate observances.

The timing framework applies: a deceased relative appearing in the fourth watch, with the dreamer waking directly to the day, carries more weight than the same appearance in the first watch, followed by return to sleep.

## Compressed Planetary Periods

Dream charts employ a compressed version of the *Viṃśottari Daśā* system scaled to a one-year cycle. The standard 120-year cycle compresses to twelve months, allowing precise timing of dream results within the maximum one-year manifestation window.

The method: identify the Moon's nakṣatra at the time of the dream. This determines the starting *daśā* lord. Calculate the proportion of the nakṣatra remaining and apply it to the compressed cycle. Subsequent planetary periods follow the standard sequence (Sun,

Moon, Mars, Rahu, Jupiter, Saturn, Mercury, Ketu, Venus) at compressed intervals.

If results do not manifest within one year, the experience did not constitute a true prophetic dream. The validation criteria hold: no luminary connection, or the dreamer returned to sleep, or the dream belonged to one of the non-prophetic categories.

## Death Dreams and the Principle of Reversal

A counterintuitive but consistent principle governs dreams of death. Varāhamihira states that dreaming of one's own death or being killed carries auspicious significance—it indicates long life, recovery from disease, and general benefit.

Similarly, dreaming of another person's death benefits that person. If one dreams of a father covered in blood while the father has a disease, the father will recover. The classical texts are consistent: dreams of death indicate benefit for the dreamed-of party.

This reversal principle echoes Egyptian paradoxical inversion. The threshold realm operates by laws contrary to waking expectation. What appears as death in the dream manifests as vitality in waking life.

One qualifier: if the dreamer kills an enemy in the dream, that enemy gains benefit. The agency shifts the outcome. And if the dead party actually dies in the dream—rather than merely being wounded—Saturn enters the picture, and the dreamer faces serious difficulty. The classical principle: the dreamed-of party should not die in the dream.

## Remediation

Here, the Vedic system shows its greatest strength. Inauspicious dreams need not manifest their negative portent. The tradition provides extensive remedial measures (*upāya*) for redirecting troubling dreams.

The underlying logic: a dream reveals conditions and tendencies, not inevitable outcomes. Appropriate action can redirect the energy. A dream is a warning and an opportunity rather than a sentence.

## *Immediate Response*

Upon waking from a disturbing dream, the dreamer should not speak of it to fools or enemies. Negative dreams told to the wrong person gain power through the telling. Instead, the dream should be reported to a learned person or priest who can provide proper remediation.

Simple acts upon waking can discharge the dream's negative charge: ritual bathing, charitable giving, recitation of specific mantras. The energy that would have manifested as an external event is redirected into ritual action.

## *Mantra*

Specific mantras address specific planetary afflictions revealed in dreams. For general protection: *Oṃ Namaḥ Śivāya* transcends ego and connects with higher consciousness. Hanumān and Durgā mantras destroy bad dreams and protect against psychic disturbance.

For lunar afflictions specifically—nightmares, emotional flooding, dreams of drowning—the invocation of Ṛṣi Atri (*Oṃ Atraye Namaḥ*) before sleep anchors the wandering *manas*. For solar afflictions—dreams of burning, exhaustion, loss of vitality—mantras to Sūrya restore the vital fire.

## *Physical Protocol*

The 90-degree leg pose—lying with feet elevated against the wall—reverses the day's downward flow of vital breath and engages the parasympathetic nervous system. Since the twelfth house is a water house, spending time near water bodies or taking soothing baths helps cleanse emotions for those with the Moon in the twelfth.

Constitutional adjustment matters. Those with excessive fire (Mars, Sun prominent in the twelfth) benefit from cooling practices—cucumber, coconut water, moonlight exposure. Those with excessive air (Rāhu, Saturn) benefit from grounding—oil massage, heavy blankets, and root vegetables.

### *The Namburbi Parallel*

This remedial technology aligns with the Mesopotamian *namburbi* rituals discussed in Chapter Three. Both traditions recognize that dreams reveal tendency, not an inevitable outcome. Diagnosis implies prognosis; prognosis enables intervention. The dream that warns is the dream that can be redirected.

The difference lies in elaboration. Mesopotamia developed ritual dissolution—transferring the portent to a substitute and destroying it. India developed a complete therapeutic system: mantric, physical, devotional, and behavioral interventions matched to the specific planetary signature revealed in the dream.

## What India Teaches

The Vedic framework advances oneiromantic practice in directions that persist through all subsequent developments.

**Validation protocol.** Not every dream warrants interpretation. The luminary connection, the broken dream principle, the sevenfold classification—these filters distinguish prophetic communication from mental noise. The practitioner who applies them wastes no time interpreting dreams that carry no weight.

**Temporal precision.** The four-watch system provides specific manifestation ranges. A fourth-watch dream manifests within days; a first-watch dream may take a year. This precision allows the practitioner to counsel appropriately: urgency for late-night dreams, patience for early-night ones.

**Planetary identification.** Dream imagery carries planetary signatures. Identifying which planet predominates allows correlation with the dreamer's natal chart and current periods. The dream of floating points to Mercury; if Mercury is afflicted natively, the dream may reveal chronic patterns rather than one-time events.

**Remedial technology.** The dream that reveals is the dream that can be redirected. India developed the most sophisticated remedial system in the oneiromantic tradition—mantras, rituals, physical practices, devotional acts matched to specific afflictions. The practitioner who understands remediation offers more than interpretation; they offer intervention.

**Karmic perspective.** Dreams may reveal patterns extending beyond this lifetime—debts from past lives seeking resolution, blessings earned through previous merit. This perspective offers both relief (the pattern is not the dreamer's fault) and direction (specific actions can address karmic debts).

## Toward the Internal Model

With the Vedic framework in place, we have surveyed the major traditions along the External-Internal Spectrum's first arc. Oral cultures recognized celestial-dream integration before writing existed. Mesopotamia systematized dream science alongside the birth of horoscopic astrology—dreams as divine messages requiring expert decoding. Egypt introduced constitutional mediation—the same dream, meaning different things for different types, the threshold becoming a colored lens. India provided validation protocols, temporal precision, and remedial technology while maintaining the fundamental premise: the dream arrives from elsewhere bearing news.

Each tradition advanced the art. Each contributed tools that the contemporary practitioner can employ. But all share a common orientation: the dream as communication *received*, whether from gods, ancestors, planets, or karmic patterns. The dreamer is the recipient. The message comes from outside.

Chinese medicine completes the spectrum by fully internalizing dream phenomena. Dreams emerge not from divine communication but from organ-spirit dynamics within the body itself. The *hún* (ethereal soul) wanders during sleep because its relationship with Liver blood requires this nocturnal activity. What appears in the dream indicates the state of internal organs, the balance of *qì*, and the condition of the Five Spirits housed in their respective *zàng*. The external has become internal. The message no longer arrives—it arises.

The three chapters that follow examine this fully internalized model: the *hún* and *pò* as dream-generating mechanisms, the Five *Shén* and their organ correspondences, and the Eight Extraordinary Vessels as the architecture through which nocturnal consciousness moves. Where India offered planetary signatures in dream content, China offers organ signatures. Where Egypt distinguished Horian from Sethian constitution, China distinguishes patterns of excess and deficiency, heat and cold, rising and sinking. The diagnostic precision rivals anything in the Western or Vedic traditions—but the ontology differs fundamentally.

We turn now to the dreaming body.

## Sources

Varāhamihira. *Bṛhat Saṃhitā*. Translated by M. Ramakrishna Bhat. Delhi: Motilal Banarsidass, 1981.

*Praśna Mārga*. Translated by B. V. Raman. Bangalore: IBH Prakashana, 1992.

*Suśruta Saṃhitā*. Translated by Kaviraj Kunjalal Bhishagratna. 3 vols. Calcutta: 1907–1916.

*Jātaka Pārijāta*. Translated by V. Subramanya Sastri. Bangalore: Raman Publications, 1966.

*Bṛhat Parāśara Horā Śāstra*. Translated by R. Santhanam. 2 vols. New Delhi: Ranjan Publications, 1984.

Rath, Sanjay. *Collected Papers in Vedic Astrology*. Vol. 1. New Delhi: Sagar Publications, 2007.

O'Flaherty, Wendy Doniger. *Dreams, Illusion, and Other Realities*. Chicago: University of Chicago Press, 1984.

# Chapter Six

# Dreaming in China: Landscape of Organ Spirits

魂之為言，如夢寐恍惚，變幻遊行之境

*Hún zhī wéi yán, rú mèngmèi huǎnghū, biànhuàn yóuxíng zhī jìng*

*"The hún in its expression is like dreaming—hazy, shifting, a realm of wandering transformation."*

—Zhang Jiebin, Lèi Jīng (Classic of Categories), 1624

Classical Chinese Medicine stands at the internal pole of the spectrum introduced in Chapter One. Where Mesopotamia received dreams as divine messages, and Egypt filtered them through a constitutional type, China locates dream origins entirely within the body. The five organ-spirits generate dream content through their nocturnal activity. What appears in sleep indicates the state of organs, the balance of *qì*, and the condition of the spirits. The external has become internal. The message no longer arrives—it arises.

## A Note on Method

Alfonso Montuori distinguishes reproductive from creative scholarship. Reproductive scholarship transmits tradition intact—faithful to sources, cautious of deviation, validated by lineage authority. Its virtue is preservation. Creative scholarship participates in tradition's evolution—faithful to the living questions that generated the sources, forging connections across domains, validated by clinical outcomes and practitioner experience. Its virtue is renewal.

This work stands in the creative mode. The *Tāng Yè Jīng* provides flavor-organ logic; Hellenistic astrology provides dignity assessment. The synthesis emerged through forty-five years of clinical attention—observing how dream quality shifts when treatment addresses planetary influences, testing whether flavor correspondences produce predicted effects. Classical sources provide vocabulary and logic; the practitioner provides integration and verification. Not doctrine—invitation.

## The Five Organ-Spirits

In Classical Chinese Medicine, consciousness is multiple—five spirits (*wǔ shén*) housed in the five *zàng* organs. Each governs distinct psychological functions; together they model the human psyche. Dreams arise when something stirs them. This framework interprets dream content and treats what dreams reveal.

The Heart's *shén* is consciousness itself—awareness, cognition, the integrating function unifying experience. The *Líng Shū* chapter "Rooted in Spirit" (*Běn Shén*) names the Heart emperor of the organ system. When *shén* is clear, the other spirits function harmoniously.

Heart-fire blazing produces agitation, insomnia, and dreams of flying or being chased. Heart-fire depleted leaves cold emptiness—spirit unhoused, wandering, unable to settle. Damp obscures *shén* differently: thinking grows muddled, foggy, slow; dreams turn murky, waterlogged, strange—confusion, suggestibility, difficulty distinguishing real from imagined.

The Liver's *hún*—ethereal soul—governs imagination, vision, life direction, the capacity for planning and dreaming. It generates a dream experience and receives extended treatment below. The Lung's *pò*—corporeal soul—enters with the first breath, governing bodily sensation, instinct, and the animal aspects of existence. The *hún* ascends and survives death; the *pò* descends and dissolves with the body. Dreams of strong physical sensation, bodily functions, or instinctual responses often arise from the *pò*. Lung pathology produces dreams of weeping, fear, flying, and white objects.

The Spleen's *yì* governs intellect, concentration, the imaginative capacity, transforming thought into action. Spleen deficiency disrupts this: difficulty focusing, obsessive rumination, paralysis of will. Dreams reveal the pattern—heaviness, sinking, inability to move, endless repetition. The Kidney's *zhì* represents willpower, determination, the drive to accomplish one's purpose—motivational force sustaining effort over time. Kidney deficiency affecting *zhì* manifests as a lack of motivation, fear, and the inability to complete projects. Dreams of water, drowning, darkness, and cold often indicate Kidney-*zhì* pathology.

*Table 6.1. Five Spirits Correspondences*

| **Organ** | **Heart** | **Liver** | **Lung** | **Spleen** | **Kidney** |
|---|---|---|---|---|---|
| Spirit | *Shén* | *Hún* | *Pò* | *Yì* | *Zhì* |
| Function | Consciousness | Vision/ Dreams | Sensation | Intellect | Willpower |
| Element | Fire | Wood | Metal | Earth | Water |
| Planet | Mars | Jupiter | Venus | Saturn | Mercury |
| Excess Dreams | Laughter, fire | Anger, fighting | Fear, flying | Singing, heaviness | Spine separating |
| Deficiency Dreams | Fire, smoke | Forests, grass | White objects | Abysses, sinking | Drowning, water |

# The Hún and the Architecture of Dreaming

The *hún* is the dream-generator. Liver, Wood, Jupiter. Among the five organ-spirits, it carries special weight—organizer of vision, strategic planning, prophetic imagery.

The relationship is reciprocal. The *Sùwèn* indicates: the Liver stores Blood; Blood houses the *hún*. Liver and *hún* shelter each other. By day, the *hún* resides in the eyes, facilitating perception and action on life's purpose. At night, it descends into the Liver to rest in the Blood.

During sleep, the *hún* separates from the body, traveling dream landscapes, contacting other beings. This wandering is the mechanism of dreaming. No wandering, no dreams. When Liver Blood is sufficient, the *hún* travels moderately, stays tethered. Dreams are vivid, coherent, and remembered. The dreamer wakes refreshed. When Blood is deficient or Liver *qì* constrained, the *hún* becomes unanchored—wanders too far, too frantically. Sleep disturbances follow: vivid or exhausting dreams, poor recall, and sleepwalking. Treatment nourishes Liver Blood. Root the wanderer; don't chase it.

Astrologically, the *hún* corresponds to Jupiter—expansion, vision, and beneficent guidance. In healthy dreaming: clear imagery, coherent narrative, prophetic insight. Jupiter holds natural affinity with the ninth house, the traditional locus of dreams and divination. Chaldean order places him there; Sagittarius, the ninth sign, is his domicile; Pisces his exaltation. Jupiter's condition in any chart—natal, dream, horary—indicates the *hún*'s capacity to generate meaningful dreams.

# Diagnostic Oneiromancy in the Yellow Emperor's Classic

*Spiritual Axis* 43, "Pathogenic Dreams," correlates dream content with organ pathology—diagnostic oneiromancy. The practitioner reads dreams as symptoms, identifying which organs require treatment. Excess and deficiency produce distinct imagery, detailed in *Simple Classic* 17 and 80.

These correlations guide diagnosis but require judgment. A water dream might indicate Kidney deficiency, or yesterday's swim. Context matters. Repetition matters. Accompanying symptoms distinguish pathology from processing. The celestial medicine practitioner adds astrological context: a water dream during Mercury's transit to natal Moon carries different significance than the same dream under Mars.

*Table 6.2. Dream Correspondences: Excess Patterns (High Dignity)*

| Phase / Planet | Zàng | Dreams |
|---|---|---|
| Wood / Jupiter | Liver | Anger, fighting, mountain forests, lying under trees |
| Fire / Mars | Heart | Laughter, fear, fire, light, mountains, smoke |
| Earth / Saturn | Spleen | Singing, heavy limbs, building houses, abyss |
| Metal / Venus | Lung | Crying, flying, worries, metal objects, white armor |
| Water / Mercury | Kidney | Fear, detachment, swimming, drowning, darkness |

*Table 6.3. Dream Correspondences: Deficiency Patterns (Low Dignity)*

| Phase / Planet | Zàng | Dreams |
|---|---|---|
| Wood / Jupiter | Liver | Mushrooms, fragrant herbs, lying in the bush |
| Fire / Mars | Heart | Volcanic eruptions, fires, heat, red objects |
| Earth / Saturn | Spleen | Hunger, marshlands, building walls, ruins |
| Metal / Venus | Lung | War, killing, white objects, strange metal shapes |
| Water / Mercury | Kidney | Plunging into water, terrifying deep sea, boats |

Sources: *Líng Shū* 4, *Sùwèn* 17, 80.

# External Versus Internal Sources

Chinese medical oneiromancy distinguishes two sources. Internal: dreams arising from organ pathology. External: genuine communications from outside the dreamer. This parallels Western categories of somatic and prophetic dreams but employs different diagnostic criteria.

Internal-source dreams correlate with other symptoms. A patient with Kidney-*zhì* deficiency dreams of drowning—and also presents with low back pain, fatigue, diminished libido, and fear. The complete picture. External-source dreams lack such correlation. The dreamer may be constitutionally robust, showing no signs of the organ pattern suggested by dream imagery. Or dream content exceeds what internal pathology could produce: specific information the dreamer could not have known, encounters with identifiable deceased persons, imagery of events that subsequently occur.

## The Tāng Yè Jīng Protocol

The *Tāng Yè Jīng* (Soup Classic), ascribed to the legendary Yi Yin, is lost—but passages survive in the *Fù Xíng Jué*, attributed to Tao Hongjing (456–536 CE). This text preserves the oldest systematic application of five-flavor therapeutics to organ pathology. Provenance is contested—addressed at the chapter's end. Clinical utility is not. Once a dream reveals an organ-spirit imbalance, the practitioner has a remediation pathway.

The five flavors—sour, bitter, sweet, pungent (aromatic), salty—each possess specific therapeutic actions, applicable to both culinary arts and herbal formula construction. The *Fù Xíng Jué* recognizes that each flavor performs different functions depending on the element treated. A flavor supplementing one organ-spirit may reduce another. The reducing flavor for one element becomes the transforming flavor for the next in the generation cycle. Supplementing (*bǔ*) addresses deficiency; reducing (*xiè*) addresses excess; transforming (*huà*) mobilizes stagnation and restores function.

## The Dignity-Flavor Paradigm

The *Tāng Yè Jīng* offers precision unavailable in standard five-phase flavor correspondences. When dream symptoms indicate organ-spirit disturbance, the astrologer differentiates based on dignity: high dignity suggests excess, middling dignity suggests stagnation, and debilitated dignity suggests depletion. This tripartite distinction guides formula selection with precision impossible under simpler models.

When dream diagnostics indicate Heart-Fire disturbance, the practitioner differentiates: reduce, supplement, or transform? Heart excess calls for bitter flavors to drain—dark leafy greens, dandelion root tea, bitter melon. Fire deficiency calls for salty flavors to nourish—miso, seaweed, bone broth with sea salt. Heart stagnation calls for sour flavors to mobilize—fermented vegetables, citrus, vinegar-dressed dishes. The *Tāng Yè Jīng* protocol completes the therapeutic arc: from dream symptom to organ-spirit diagnosis to daily nourishment.

*Table 6.4. Flavor Actions by Planet*

| **Planet** | **Mercury** | **Venus** | **Mars** | **Jupiter** | **Saturn** |
|---|---|---|---|---|---|
| Phase | Water | Metal | Fire | Wood | Earth |
| Organ | Kidney | Lung | Heart | Liver | Spleen |
| Spirit | Zhì | Pò | Shén | Hún | Yì |
| Transforms | Salty | Aromatic | Sour | Sweet | Bitter |
| Reduces | Sweet | Salty | Bitter | Sour | Aromatic |
| Supplements | Bitter | Sour | Salty | Aromatic | Sweet |

Therapeutic action follows planetary dignity—the root of this integration. High dignity (domicile, exaltation, strong triplicity): the organ-spirit functions robustly, potentially to excess. The reducing flavor drains surplus. Low dignity (detriment, fall, peregrine): the organ-spirit is depleted. The supplementing flavor nourishes. Slow movement or neutral dignity: stagnation. The transforming flavor mobilizes and restores function.

Jupiter. Wood. Liver. The *hún*—transcendent soul. When Jupiter is dignified, and anger dreams or excessive wandering indicate overactivity, sourness reduces. When Jupiter is debilitated, and deficiency dreams of forests and grass reveal depletion, aromatic supplements are recommended. When Jupiter is neutral or slow-moving, sweet transforms—mobilizing stagnant Liver *qì*, restoring the *hún*'s capacity for vision. Jupiter and the *hún* govern dream-generating capacity. These flavors address dream quality at its source.

# The Ninth House and the Five Visible Planets

In celestial medicine dream work, the ninth house commands attention. The ninth governs dreams, prophecy, and divine communication. The Almuten—the strongest influencing planet on the ninth cusp from among the five visible planets—indicates the dreamer's access to these realms. Since each visible planet corresponds to an organ-spirit and its associated flavors, the *Tāng Yè Jīng* protocol applies directly. Improving dream quality and treating the organ-spirit become one intervention.

Jupiter remains relevant regardless of which planet holds the ninth cusp—his natural affinity with dreams and the *hún* makes him perpetual significator. Assessment is twofold: the ninth house Almuten indicates which organ-spirit most shapes prophetic access; Jupiter's own condition indicates baseline dream-generating capacity. The practice brings both together—the flavor of the ninth Almuten combined with the flavor supporting Jupiter. When Jupiter is well-dignified, the ethereal soul functions robustly; debilitated, dream quality suffers, and Liver-*hún* pathology underlies.

# Two Methods for Formula Construction

Two methods translate the *Tāng Yè Jīng* protocol into clinical practice.

***Method One: Jupiter's Dignities.*** Since the *hún* is the dream-generator, Jupiter's condition in the horary chart guides treatment. Cast a chart for the moment the dream is reported. Identify every planet ruling Jupiter's position by domicile, exaltation, triplicity, term, and face. Each visible planet among these contributes its organ-spirit to the assessment. Jupiter's overall dignity determines the therapeutic action: high dignity calls for the reducing flavor; low dignity calls for the supplementing flavor; neutral or slow-moving calls for the transforming flavor. The method addresses all planetary influences on the *hún*'s condition simultaneously.

***Method Two: The Term Ruler of the Ninth Cusp.*** A more direct approach focuses on the ninth house cusp itself. Since terms divide each sign into five segments ruled by different planets, the term ruler of the ninth cusp indicates which organ-spirit most immediately shapes prophetic access. Assess this planet's dignity, then apply the corresponding flavor action. Always check Jupiter as well—if the *hún* itself is compromised, address both.

Worked examples with full dignity calculations and culinary applications appear in Appendix E.

## Dosage and Timing

Spirit doses—drop doses of tincture, pinch doses of powder—suffice for soul-level treatment. The formula's power lies in coherence, not quantity. Administer during planetary hours aligned with intention. For *hún*-level treatment, use Jupiter hours. For dream quality specifically, the hour of the ninth house ruler. When addressing a specific planet's influence on the *hún*, use that planet's hour.

## Unity of the Five Spirits

Health is harmony among the five organ-spirits. The model ascends through the generating cycle. Water is the root. Kidney will (*zhì*), firm in purpose, nourishes the Liver ethereal soul (*hún*). The *hún*, rooted and ranging, nourishes Heart spirit (*shén*). When *shén* is clear, it nourishes Spleen consciousness (*yì*). When *yì* is steady, it nourishes Lung corporeal soul (*pò*). When *pò* is grounded, it completes the circuit.

When this cycle flows unobstructed, the human being functions as a coherent whole. Dreams arising from such a state are clear, meaningful, and restorative.

The Organ Gaze practice cultivates this harmony directly. Generate a soft smile—genuine, felt in the eyes. Let this warmth descend through the body, following the generating cycle:

*Kidneys:* Fear softens. *Zhì* steadies. Water roots.

*Liver:* Anger releases. *Hún* settles. Wood grows from Water.

*Heart:* Anxiety calms. *Shén* clarifies. Fire rises from Wood.

*Spleen:* Worry dissolves. *Yì* grounds. Earth receives Fire's ash.

*Lungs:* Grief eases. *Pò* anchors. Metal condenses from Earth.

Each organ holds characteristic emotional residue. The smile does not suppress—it transforms. Attention plus warmth plus time. Done regularly, the practice clears obstructions before they manifest as pathology—preventive dream medicine. The organ-spirits, harmonized by day, produce coherent dreams by night.

## Synthesis

The dream diagnoses; the chart quantifies; the flavors treat. Through this threefold method, the practitioner addresses soul-level disturbance at its root. Jupiter and the *hún* govern dream-generating capacity; the ninth house Almuten and term ruler identify which organ-spirit shapes prophetic access; the *Tāng Yè Jīng* protocol translates diagnosis into daily nourishment. The five organ-spirits, attended to through food and planetary timing, return to natural harmony. Dreams clarify. The wanderer comes home.

This is medicine for dreams that arise from within—organ-spirits stirring, the *hún* wandering according to its nature, the body speaking in the only language sleep allows. Flavor and timing redirect; balance restores; the dreamer wakes refreshed.

But not all dream disturbance arises from within. Sometimes the *hún* wanders too far and encounters what it should not. Sometimes something enters while defenses sleep. The dreamer wakes exhausted, depleted, as if something fed on them during the night. Classical Chinese Medicine names this pattern directly: dreams of intercourse with ghosts. The following chapter examines this territory—where psychological boundary dissolves, where fixation takes up residence, and where the architecture of anchoring becomes medicine's most urgent task.

# A Note on the Tāng Yè Jīng and Fù Xíng Jué

The five-flavor therapeutics derive from the *Fù Xíng Jué*, attributed to Tao Hongjing (456–536 CE), claiming to preserve passages from the lost *Tāng Yè Jīng*, ascribed to the legendary Yi Yin.

Provenance is contested. The *Fù Xíng Jué* emerged publicly in 1974 when Zhang Dachang, a Hebei village physician, presented a hand-copy to the Chinese Academy of Traditional Chinese Medicine—his grandfather had purchased the original silk scroll from Wang Yuanlu, discoverer of the Dunhuang Library Cave, in 1918. That original was reportedly destroyed during the Cultural Revolution. Suspicion of forgery followed. Scholars divide: Zhang Zhenglang and Li Xueqin concluded it was neither an authentic early composition nor a modern fabrication; Ma Jixing, Qian Chaochen, and Wang Xuetai argued for antiquity; Tian Yongyan argued against.

Archival debates are not the final word. Family lineages continue employing this framework—living traditions validating through generations of clinical use. The *Tǐ-Yòng-Huà* paradigm, the flavor-organ correspondences—these appear nowhere else yet cohere as functional methodology. Content, consistency, clinical efficacy validate a medical text. Not archival certainty. The *Huáng Dì Nèi Jīng* and *Shāng Hán Lùn* lack original manuscripts. No one dismisses them as fabrications.

# Sources

Fruehauf, Heiner. "The Fu Xing Jue: An Ancient Source Text on the Constitutional Treatment of the Five Organ Networks." Classical Chinese Medicine. Accessed 2024. https://classicalchinesemedicine.org.

*Huángdì Nèijīng Líng Shū*. Translated by Paul Unschuld. Berkeley: University of California Press, 2016.

*Huángdì Nèijīng Sùwèn*. Translated by Paul Unschuld and Hermann Tessenow. Berkeley: University of California Press, 2011.

Ma Jixing. *Dunhuang Guyiji Kaoshi* [Research on Ancient Medical Texts from Dunhuang]. Nanchang: Jiangxi Kexue Jishu Chubanshe, 1988.

Maciocia, Giovanni. *The Psyche in Chinese Medicine*. Edinburgh: Churchill Livingstone, 2009.

Montuori, Alfonso. "The Complexity of Transdisciplinarity: A Review of Basarab Nicolescu's Manifesto of Transdisciplinarity." *Metanexus*, 2005.

Qian Chaochen. "Textual Research on the Fuxing Jue." *Zhonghua Yishi Zazhi* [Chinese Journal of Medical History] 18, no. 2 (1988): 69–76.

Wang Xuetai. "Studies on the Fuxing Jue Zangfu Yongyao Fayao." *Zhongguo Zhongyi Jichu Yixue Zazhi* [Chinese Journal of Basic Medicine in Traditional Chinese Medicine] 5, no. 3 (1999): 52–55.

## Chapter Seven

# Spirit Disturbance and the Ghostly Dream

鬼交之病，神不守舍

*Guǐ jiāo zhī bìng, shén bù shǒu shè*

*"The illness of ghostly intercourse:*
*the spirit does not guard its dwelling."*

—Chao Yuanfang, Zhūbìng Yuánhòu Lùn
(Treatise on the Origins and Symptoms of Disease), 610 CE

# The Ghost in the Bedroom

Classical Chinese Medicine names a clinical pattern: dreams of intercourse with ghosts. The *Essentials from the Golden Cabinet* (circa 220 CE) is the earliest surviving medical text to formalize this diagnosis.

The chapter on excessive action bringing depletion distinguishes manifestation by gender: in men, depletion appears as nocturnal emissions without dreaming; in women, as dreaming of intercourse with ghosts. For both, the text prescribes Cinnamon Twig Decoction plus Dragon Bone and Oyster Shell.

The formula addresses fragmentation of self—leakage of essence (*jīng*) alongside destabilization of spirit (*shén*). The ghost is diagnostic language: mental fixations, addictions, erosion of psychological boundaries. What haunts modern patients' sleep.

The concept circulated beyond medical literature. Daoist texts warned that improper sexual practices could lead to "the illness of copulation with ghosts." Ge Hong's *Zhǒuhòu Fāng* (*Handbook of Formulas for Emergencies*, circa 340 CE) expanded the discussion—both men and women might dream of intercourse with human beings or demons, treatable by herbal prescription, acupuncture, and moxibustion.

The term *ghostly intercourse* marks a state where boundaries have become porous. Something gets in. Something gets out. By the Song Dynasty, medical literature elaborated: such dreams were movements of *shén*-spirits—literal components of the body that had wandered away or been intruded upon by external pathogenic *qì*. The ghost might be ancestor, demon, or *húlí jīng*—the fox spirit who cultivates power over centuries, shapeshifts into human form, enters the dreamer's bed to drain essence through seduction.

Foxes, snakes, weasels: shapeshifters crossing the boundary between animal and human, wild and domestic, predator and prey. This is shamanic territory inverted. The shaman journeys outward, negotiates with spirits, retrieves what was lost. The shapeshifter journeys inward—into the sleeper, into the body, into the unguarded night. Clinical meaning did not vary: something feeding while you sleep.

## The Twelfth House and the Bedroom

Western astrology locates these experiences in the twelfth house—the place of self-undoing, hidden enemies, confinement. And the bedroom. Traditional texts call it *cacodaemon*, "bad spirit," where planets lose capacity for effective action. What happens in the twelfth happens in darkness, hidden from public view and often from the native's own awareness.

The bedroom is twelfth-house territory. Sleep is the most constantly needed bedroom pleasure—more fundamental than sex, more nightly than love. Dreams follow. Then the rest: intimacy, vulnerability, what we do when no one watches. The twelfth governs all of it. Ghosts enter through this house. So do lovers. The threshold makes no moral distinction. It marks the boundary between waking agency and nocturnal surrender.

Planets in the twelfth operate strangely. Significations become diffuse, hard to grasp, prone to manifest through dreams, fantasies, and projections. Venus in the twelfth: secret loves, hidden pleasures, erotic imagination exceeding what daylight relationships contain. Mars in the twelfth: anger finding no direct outlet, aggression turned inward or expressed through passive means, sexual energy operating underground. Saturn in the twelfth: fears one cannot name, sorrows carried in isolation, the weight of what remains unprocessed.

The twelfth-house ghost is the visitor arriving when ego sleeps. In Chinese medical terms, this is *hún* territory—the ethereal soul wandering beyond the body's boundaries, encountering what it encounters. When Liver Blood is deficient and the *hún* cannot anchor properly, these encounters become pathological. The ghost takes up residence. The dreamer wakes exhausted, depleted, as if something fed on them during the night.

Assessment requires examining both the twelfth house and Jupiter, the *hún*'s planetary correlate. Afflictions to the twelfth—malefics present, ruler debilitated or under hard aspect—indicate vulnerability to intrusion. Jupiter's condition indicates whether the *hún* can maintain coherence during nocturnal wandering. When both are compromised, the bedroom becomes haunted ground.

# The Architecture of Anchoring

Cinnamon Twig Decoction plus Dragon Bone and Oyster Shell modifies Cinnamon Twig Decoction, the first formula of the *Treatise on Cold Damage*. By adding two heavy, mineral-based substances—Dragon Bone (*Fossilia Ossis Mastodi,* Lóng Gǔ) and Oyster Shell (*Ostrea gigas* shell, Mǔ Lì)—Zhang Zhongjing transformed a formula for harmonizing the exterior (*yíng* and *wèi* levels) into one capable of anchoring the deep interior.

Both substances are calcium-rich. Modern reductionism stops there—calcium supplementation, nothing more. But fossils and shells carry more than elemental chemistry. Dragon Bone is fossilized mammal bone, often millions of years old, mineralized under pressure over geological time. Oyster Shell forms through the living process of a creature building its protective enclosure, layer by layer, from the ocean. One derives from ancient land animals, the other from contemporary sea creatures. One represents time compressed into mineral density; the other represents the ocean's capacity to precipitate structure from dissolved salts.

The clinical effects exceed what calcium alone could produce. Calcium supplements do not anchor the *shén*. They do not stop night sweats, calm palpitations, or prevent seminal emission. Dragon Bone and Oyster Shell do. The difference lies in what Chinese medicine calls *qì*—the organizational pattern carried by the substance, not merely its molecular constituents. The fossil carries the pattern of deep time, of substance that has endured. The shell carries the pattern of protective enclosure, of boundaries formed against the flux of water. These patterns communicate to the body's own organizing intelligence. The *shén* receives the message: settle, consolidate, hold firm.

*Table 7.1. Composition of Cinnamon Twig Decoction plus Dragon Bone and Oyster Shell*

| Ingredient | Pharmaceutical Name | Traditional Function |
|---|---|---|
| *Cinnamomum cassia* twig (Guì Zhī) | Cinnamomi Ramulus | Warms yang; opens exterior; harmonizes yíng and wèi |
| *Paeonia lactiflora* root (Bái Sháo) | Paeoniae Radix Alba | Nourishes Blood; restrains yin; consolidates interior |
| Dragon Bone (Lóng Gǔ) | Fossilia Ossis Mastodi | Anchors spirit; astringes essence; settles Liver |
| *Ostrea gigas* shell (Mǔ Lì) | Ostreae Concha | Subdues yang; softens hardness; stabilizes Heart-Kidney axis |
| *Zingiber officinale* rhizome (Shēng Jiāng) | Zingiberis Rhizoma Recens | Harmonizes the Stomach; assists yang circulation |
| *Ziziphus jujuba* fruit (Dà Zǎo) | Jujubae Fructus | Tonifies qì; nourishes Blood; cushions spirit |
| *Glycyrrhiza uralensis* root (Gān Cǎo) | Glycyrrhizae Radix | Harmonizes all herbs; tonifies the middle |

The base formula balances the ascending, warming nature of Cinnamon Twig (*Cinnamomum cassia* twig, Guì Zhī) against the descending, nourishing nature of White Peony (*Paeonia lactiflora* root, Bái Sháo). This is the formula's pivot—the Cinnamon-Peony balance governing psychological boundaries, detailed in the closing section below.

When this rhythm destabilizes—too much opening, insufficient holding—the boundary becomes porous. Something gets in. Something gets out. The ghost enters through the gap. In cases of profound deficiency taxation where *yáng* floats and *yīn* is exhausted, this harmonization alone is insufficient. Dragon Bone and Oyster Shell serve as weight to pull the pivot downward into the Heart and Kidney channels.

Dragon Bone enters the Kidney channel, restraining essence and preventing leakage of *jīng*. Oyster Shell enters the Heart channel, settling rising *yáng* and cooling empty fire that agitates the mind. Together, they rectify the relationship between Heart (Fire) and

Kidney (Water). In health, Kidney water ascends to cool Heart fire while Heart fire descends to warm Kidney water. When this axis breaks, Heart fire flares upward, causing dream-disturbed sleep and palpitations, while Kidney essence leaks downward, causing spermatorrhea or vaginal discharge.

## The Ghost as Euphemism

Classical Chinese thought blurred the literal ghost and the psychological state. Dreams were the wandering of *hún*. When *qì* and Blood ran deficient, the *hún* lost its tether and wandered into realms where it encountered ghosts. As medical tradition matured through Tang and Song, physicians like Sun Simiao began using ghost language metaphorically—heavy emotional disturbance, mental confusion, what we cannot shake off.

Dreams of intercourse with ghosts are a euphemism. The ghost is an intrusive thought. Fixated memory. Desire that will not release. A presence haunting consciousness, detached from the present moment, feeding on attention.

## The Hungry Ghost and Addiction

The Buddhist concept of the *Preta* or Hungry Ghost—entities with pinhole necks and giant bellies who can never be satisfied—is the standard metaphor for addiction. The formula is frequently used in contemporary practice for drug withdrawal and cravings, anchoring frantic, grasping *yáng* energy that drives addictive behavior. Patients who dream of ghosts often exhibit psychological boundary issues: inability to say no, tendency to absorb emotions of others, feeling possessed by one's own impulses or expectations of others.

In later imperial China, medical texts associated dreams of ghostly intercourse with sexual frustration, madness, and demonic fetuses (false pregnancies). The ghost contained desires or traumas socially or personally unacceptable, emerging in the dream state when conscious defensive *qì* was low.

## The Mechanism of Spirit Fragmentation

The formula's effectiveness depends on the relationship between two souls described in Chapter Six. When Kidney *jīng* depletes, the corporeal soul (*pò*) escapes governance of the ethereal soul (*hún*). The ghost in the dream is *pò* unmoored—acting out primal drives for sex, food, safety without mediation from higher spirits. Dragon Bone and Oyster Shell anchor the *pò*, restore hierarchy, and return it to governance of *hún* and *shén*.

## Modern Clinical Indications

Clinical presentation spans physical sexual dysfunction to advanced neurosis. The underlying pattern: interior deficiency with floating *yáng*—empty inside, agitated above. In astrological terms: essential debility with accidental dignity, or a peregrine planet in an angular house. Weak foundation, prominent expression. Modern practitioners have expanded the formula's use to include PTSD and trauma, particularly sexual abuse, where the ghost of trauma continues to violate the person's psychological space during sleep.

*Table 7.2. Clinical Indications by Domain*

| Domain | Symptoms | Pathophysiology |
|---|---|---|
| Reproductive | Spermatorrhea, premature ejaculation, impotence, frigidity, cold genitals | Kidney yang failing to restrain fluids; essence leaking due to floating Heart fire |
| Psychological | Anxiety, panic attacks, irritability, emotional instability, boundary issues | Heart-Kidney disharmony; unanchored shén with hyper-reactivity |
| Neurological | Insomnia, sexual dreams, dizziness, palpitations, forgetfulness | Liver Blood deficiency failing to anchor hún; empty heat agitating mind |
| Constitutional | Hair loss, diarrhea, cold extremities, abdominal tension, hollow pulse | Profound vacuity taxation; yīn and yáng failing to interpenetrate |

The formula treats mental agitation and drug ideation during withdrawal from methamphetamines or opioids. It addresses the erratic complaints syndrome (*xuè dào zhèng*), where symptoms shift frequently, reflecting a lack of internal containment.

# Contemporary Pharmacological Mechanisms

Pharmacological research confirms what tradition observed. The formula normalizes the HPA axis—the stress-response system hyperactive in chronic anxiety and depression. It inhibits inflammatory cytokines (IL-1β, IL-6, TNF-α), reducing neuroinflammation that clouds perception. In traditional terms: clearing phlegm from the portals of the *shén*.

The sedative effects work through neurotransmission. Licorice (*Glycyrrhiza uralensis* root, Gān Cǎo) modulates GABA and serotonin receptors. Dragon Bone and Oyster Shell influence calcium channels—the molecular basis for their anchoring action on the nervous system. Calcium governs nerve impulse and muscle tone. The minerals stabilize at the cellular level what tradition describes as settling the spirit.

Recent studies show the formula promotes neuronal repair—autophagy, synaptic plasticity, activation of healing pathways. Chronic stress damages neurons; the formula helps restore them. Biochemical restoration mirrors traditional action: astringing essence, consolidating the interior, rebuilding boundaries at every level. See Appendix G for detailed neurochemistry.

# Reclaiming the Spirit from the Ghostly Realm

Cinnamon Twig Decoction plus Dragon Bone and Oyster Shell demonstrates the psychological sophistication of early Chinese medicine. The most intimate ghostly encounters are manifestations of unanchored desires and depleted boundaries. Eighteen hundred years ago, the

*Essentials from the Golden Cabinet* offered a path to reintegration. It remains open.

The formula's architecture rests on a single pivot: the relationship between Cinnamon Twig (*Cinnamomum cassia* twig, Guì Zhī) and White Peony (*Paeonia lactiflora* root, Bái Sháo). Cinnamon opens outward—warming, dispersing, moving *qì* from interior to exterior, activating the body's defensive boundary with the world. White Peony draws inward—cooling, consolidating, nourishing Blood and restraining *yīn*, anchoring awareness in the interior. Together they establish the psyche's fundamental oscillation: engagement and withdrawal, expression and containment, reaching out and pulling back. When this rhythm destabilizes—too much opening, insufficient holding—the boundary becomes porous. Something gets in. Something gets out. The ghost enters through the gap.

Dragon Bone (*Fossilia Ossis Mastodi,* Lóng Gǔ) and Oyster Shell (*Ostrea gigas* shell, Mǔ Lì) add weight to this dynamic, pulling the pivot downward into Kidney and Heart. They do not replace the Cinnamon-Peony balance; they anchor it. The formula treats boundary failure at every level: skin and muscle (the *yíng-wèi* interface), psyche and world (the capacity to say no), consciousness and unconsciousness (the threshold crossed nightly in sleep).

The Indian tradition names what the Chinese call "ghost" with different precision. *Saṃskāra*—the accumulated impressions of past action, the grooves worn into consciousness by repeated experience, the residue of *karma* manifesting as mental tendency. Every addiction is *saṃskāra.* Every compulsion. Every pattern that runs without conscious consent. The ghost feeding while you sleep is *saṃskāra* activated in the absence of waking vigilance—old patterns replaying, old hungers reasserting, old wounds reopening in the vulnerable hours.

*Saṃskāra* explains why the ghost returns. Treat the depletion, anchor the spirit, restore the boundary—and still the pattern may reassert when conditions align. The formula addresses the terrain; awareness addresses the visitor. Without herbal support, awareness lacks a stable ground. Without awareness, herbs can only suppress what will eventually resurface. The treatment is both: consolidate the *jīng,* anchor the *shén*, and simultaneously bring consciousness to what has operated in darkness.

This is why the formula alone does not cure trauma. It creates conditions for integration. The ghost must be met—not with the scattered attention of depletion, but with the consolidated presence the formula provides. Dragon Bone and Oyster Shell settle the spirit so that what was intolerable can finally be witnessed. Cinnamon Twig warms the *yáng* so the psyche can engage rather than collapse. White Peony nourishes the Blood so the *hún* has somewhere to return. The architecture supports the encounter. The encounter transforms the *saṃskāra*.

Modern presentations require this understanding. Spermatorrhea or trauma survival—the core action is the same. Stop the leakage of essence. Anchor the wandering soul. But add: *bring awareness to what feeds in the dark*.

Digital fixations. Fragmented attention. Doom-scrolling at 2 a.m. The compulsive reach for a phone, drink, or drug. The lingering presence of an abuser visiting dreams decades later. Loss of focus. Loss of vitality. These are *saṃskāra* in contemporary dress—grooves worn so deep they run automatically, ghosts so familiar we mistake them for self.

The formula treats the whole person—body, *qì*, spirit. *Shén* settles. *Hún* roots. *Pò* returns to governance. The Cinnamon-Peony pivot restores the psyche's capacity to open and close, engage and withdraw, meet the world and return to center. The mineral weight of Dragon Bone and Oyster Shell provides ballast against the pull of old patterns. Turbulence quiets. Instincts anchor. Traumatic memories integrate rather than intrude.

The ghost, named and treated, dissolves. What remains is not absence but presence—the self consolidated, aware, capable of meeting what arises without being consumed. The boundary holds. The spirit guards its dwelling. Sleep becomes restoration rather than predation.

# The Thirteen Ghost Points

While Cinnamon Twig Decoction plus Dragon Bone and Oyster Shell addresses the ghost through herbal harmonization, Classical Chinese Medicine also employs the Thirteen Ghost Points, developed by Sun Simiao in the seventh century. These points treat spirit disturbance and what was historically termed possession—now understood as severe mental illness, mania, or deep-seated trauma. The concept of ghost (*guǐ*) in this context is synonymous with excess phlegm, the medium allowing malevolent spirits or fixations to take residence in the body.

The points need not be needled. Touch activates them. So do gems placed on the skin—clear quartz to clarify *shén*, black tourmaline to ground and protect, amethyst to calm agitation. Crystals carry mineral signatures similar to Dragon Bone and Oyster Shell: anchoring, stabilizing, communicating structure to scattered spirit. Essential oils applied to ghost points extend the treatment: frankincense for Du 26 (Ghost Palace) to clear the mind, lavender for Pc 7 (Ghost Heart) to calm anxiety, vetiver for St 6 (Ghost Bed) to ground and root.

Use a reference for point locations such as Peter Deadman's *A Manual of Acupuncture*. Training in these methods is essential.

*Table 7.3. The Thirteen Ghost Points*

*First Trinity: Beginning of psychological dysfunction; phlegm blocking the orifices; wandering shén*

| Point | Ghost Name | Indication |
|---|---|---|
| Du 26 | Ghost Palace (Guǐ Gōng) | Revives consciousness; clears mind during emotional shock; ancestral trauma |
| Lu 11 | Ghost Faith (Guǐ Xìn) | Releases stagnant Lung energy; aids letting go of grief; broken vows |
| Sp 1 | Ghost Fortress (Guǐ Lěi) | Grounds the spirit; treats obsessive thinking; eating disorders |

*Second Trinity: Wind causing excess movement or paralysis; inflexible attitudes; no life direction*

| Point | Ghost Name | Indication |
|---|---|---|
| Pc 7 | Ghost Heart (Guǐ Xīn) | Calms the Heart; releases deeply held emotional pain; broken relationships |
| Bl 62 | Ghost Road (Guǐ Lù) | Opens the Yang Qiao Mai; treats insomnia, epilepsy; wandering at night |
| Du 16 | Ghost Pillow (Guǐ Zhěn) | Clears wind from the brain; treats mania, headaches, stiff neck |

*Third Trinity: Addiction; the patient is stuck using stimulants; the ghost has fully taken hold*

| Point | Ghost Name | Indication |
|---|---|---|
| St 6 | Ghost Bed (Guǐ Chuáng) | Treats PTSD, addiction; loss of empathy; lockjaw, Bell's palsy, epilepsy |
| Ren 24 | Ghost Market (Guǐ Shì) | Dark thoughts, deep depression; the ghost absorbs the yīn; no smile |
| Pc 8 | Ghost Cave (Guǐ Kū) | Lost sense of self; paranoia, self-destruction; pattern at nutritive level |

*Fourth Trinity: The ghost has moved into the deepest levels; patient's health demises*

| Point | Ghost Name | Indication |
|---|---|---|
| Du 23 | Ghost Hall (Guǐ Táng) | Clears the brain; treats nasal obstruction, dizziness, severe anxiety |
| Ren 1 | Ghost Store (Guǐ Cáng) | Treats collapse of yáng; loss of consciousness; resuscitation point |
| LI 11 | Ghost Leg (Guǐ Chén) | Clears heat; treats high fever with delirium; paralysis of upper limbs |

*Thirteenth Point: The seal*

| Point | Ghost Name | Indication |
|---|---|---|
| Haiquan (MHN-37) | Ghost Seal (Guǐ Fēng) | Under the tongue; reconnects Du and Ren; schizophrenia, loss of speech |

The Four Trinities represent the progression of possession—the ghost's deepening hold on the person. Early stages (First Trinity) show wandering *shén* and initial psychological dysfunction. Later stages (Fourth Trinity) represent complete takeover, the person no longer recognizable as themselves. Treatment proceeds according to depth of invasion.

Use of these points alongside formulas like Cinnamon Twig Decoction plus Dragon Bone and Oyster Shell offers a comprehensive strategy for reclaiming oneself from fixations occupying the Ghost Bed of the mind.

The following chapter turns to Daoist tradition, where the twelfth house offers yet another lens for reading the architecture of sleep and dream.

## Sources


Bensky, Dan, Steven Clavey, and Erich Stöger. *Chinese Herbal Medicine: Formulas and Strategies*. 2nd ed. Seattle: Eastland Press, 2009.

Bensky, Dan, Steven Clavey, and Erich Stöger. *Chinese Herbal Medicine: Materia Medica*. 3rd ed. Seattle: Eastland Press, 2004.

Chao Yuanfang. *Zhūbìng Yuánhòu Lùn* (Treatise on the Origins and Symptoms of Disease). 610 CE.

Deadman, Peter, Mazin Al-Khafaji, and Kevin Baker. *A Manual of Acupuncture*. Hove, East Sussex: Journal of Chinese Medicine Publications, 1998.

Ge Hong. *Zhǒuhòu Fāng* (Handbook of Formulas for Emergencies). Circa 340 CE.

Robinet, Isabelle. *Taoism: Growth of a Religion*. Stanford: Stanford University Press, 1997.

Sun Simiao. *Bèi Jí Qiān Jīn Yào Fāng* (Essential Prescriptions Worth a Thousand Gold). 7th century CE.

Zhang Zhongjing. *Jīn Guì Yào Lüè* (Essentials from the Golden Cabinet). Circa 220 CE.

# Chapter Eight

# Daoist Sleep Cultivation

真人本無睡，睡則浮雲煙

*Zhēn rén běn wú shuì, shuì zé fú yún yān*

*"Realized Ones are fundamentally without sleep;*
*when they sleep, they float on mist and clouds."*

—Chen Tuan, Lì Shuì Shī
(Poem on Encouraging the Sleeping Gong)

## From Healing to Path

The preceding chapters addressed dreams as diagnostic phenomena. This chapter shifts register. Sleep becomes practice. The goal is not interpretation but transformation—not healing but return.

Liu Ming organized dream work into three progressive layers: Healing, Divination, and Path. This chapter concerns the third.

Most people never move beyond the first layer. They manage sleep problems, extract occasional insight from memorable dreams, and consider the matter settled. But contemplative traditions recognize that nightly dissolution of waking consciousness opens a door. What lies beyond—and how to pass through deliberately—is the subject of this chapter.

The Daoist tradition calls this practice *Shuì Gōng* (睡功): Sleeping Cultivation. The techniques trace to Chen Tuan (d. 989 CE), a sage who lived on Mount Hua and became known as the Sleeping Immortal for his ability to remain in meditative sleep for extended periods, emerging refreshed and radiant. His methods were not mere rest. They were technology for returning consciousness to its source.

That source, in Daoist terminology, is the Pre-Celestial state (*Xiāntiān*)—existence before differentiation, before polarity, before the fragmentation characterizing ordinary waking life. Every spiritual tradition names this primordial unity. *Ein Sof* in Kabbalah. *Brahman* in Vedanta. The *Pleroma* in Gnostic Christianity. The One of Neoplatonism. Names differ; referent is the same. *Shuì Gōng* provides a method for accessing this state through the natural gateway of sleep.

## Basic Cosmology

Understanding *Shuì Gōng* requires orientation to Daoist cosmology. The framework is simple; its implications unfold across a lifetime.

Before differentiation—if "before" applies outside time—there is only undifferentiated potential. The Daoists call this *Wújí*, the

Limitless: an empty circle. Not nothing, but everything in potential before anything becomes actual. Luminous emptiness.

Movement stirs within stillness. Polarity emerges: *Yang* (light, expansion, activity) and *Yin* (dark, contraction, rest). This first differentiation is *Tàijí*, the Great Pole—the familiar symbol of interlocking dark and light.

From polarity, further differentiation. The Five Agents emerge: Wood, Fire, Earth, Metal, Water. From the Five Agents, the Ten Thousand Things of manifest existence.

This manifest world is *Hòutiān*, the Post-Celestial state: birth and death, gain and loss, time and change. Every human being enters *Hòutiān* at first breath. Before that—in the womb—the fetus exists closer to *Xiāntiān*, the Pre-Celestial: sustained by the mother's vitality, not yet breathing independently, not yet fully separate.

The ordinary direction of life moves from unity toward fragmentation, vitality toward depletion. But Daoist alchemists discovered that this direction can be reversed. The practitioner traces the path backward: multiplicity toward unity, depletion toward vitality, Ten Thousand Things toward the undifferentiated source.

This reversal is the essence of internal alchemy (*Nèidān*). The maxim states: "Those who follow the ordinary course give birth to human beings; those who reverse it become immortals."

Sleep provides an opportunity for reversal. Every night, waking consciousness naturally dissolves. The discriminating mind releases its grip. For the unprepared, this produces only ordinary unconsciousness. For the practitioner who navigates this threshold deliberately, sleep becomes a gate to the source.

## The Reversal of the Five Agents

The ordinary sequence of the Five Agents proceeds: Wood generates Fire, Fire generates Earth, Earth generates Metal, Metal generates Water, Water generates Wood. This is the *shēng* cycle—each phase giving rise to the next. In the human being, this governs the flow from birth toward death.

The alchemical reversal traces the sequence backward. Fire returns to Wood. Earth returns to Fire. The child returns to the mother. This backward movement is *nì*—reversal, inversion—the fundamental operation of internal alchemy.

The ordinary direction scatters. The reversal gathers. The Five Agents do not cease to exist; they cease to exist separately. Their distinct energies merge into the single primordial breath from which they emerged. The *Nèidān* texts call this the gathering of the Five Forces at the Source (*Wǔ Qì Cháo Yuán*): fragmentation resolving into unity.

In *Shuì Gōng*, this gathering occurs through stillness. The waking activities that scatter the Five Agents—seeing and planning (Wood), excitement and agitation (Fire), thinking and worrying (Earth), grieving and letting go (Metal), fearing and efforting (Water)—all cease. The organs rest. The emotions settle. The scattered forces return toward the center.

## Organ Gazing

The practice of directing awareness through the internal organs traces to the *Neiguan* (Inner Observation) tradition formalized in the Tang dynasty. In sleep cultivation, this organ-directed awareness follows the reversal sequence, gathering each energy back to its source.

Generate a soft awareness—genuine, felt in the eyes—and direct this warmth through the organs in reverse sequence.

Begin at the Kidneys. Awareness descends to the lower back. Fear softens; *zhì* (will) steadies. Water consolidates at its source. Rest until the Kidneys feel full, quiet, and settled.

Move to the Lungs. Water receives Metal back into itself. Awareness suffuses the chest; grief eases; *pò* (corporeal soul) grounds.

Move to the Spleen. Earth returns to Metal. Awareness settles in the center; worry dissolves; *yì* (intellect) quiets.

Move to the Heart. Fire returns to Earth. Awareness warms the chest; agitation calms; *shén* (spirit) clarifies.

Move to the Liver. Wood returns to Fire. Awareness suffuses the right side beneath the ribs; anger releases; *hún* (ethereal soul) roots. The eyes soften, the planning mind releases.

Return to the Kidneys. The circle completes—not the ordinary generating circle but the reverse, the gathering circle. All five energies are gathered in the lower belly, below the navel. Not as five but as one. Awareness dissolves into this unity. The practitioner rests at the source.

## The Gate of the Mysterious Female

At the center of this practice lies what the *Dàodé Jīng* calls the Gate of the Mysterious Female (*Xuán Pìn Zhī Mén*):

> *The Spirit of the Valley is immortal and is called the Mysterious Feminine. This Womb of the Universe is the Gate at the root of Heaven and Earth. Flowing softly and continuously, it seems to exist. Use it; it is never exhausted.* —*Dàodé Jīng*, Chapter 6

The true Gate has no fixed physical location—"neither inside nor outside" the body. It cannot be found by searching. It reveals itself when conditions are right.

The Mysterious (*xuán*) represents *Yang*; the Female (*pìn*) represents *Yin*. The character *pìn* carries the meaning of womb—the Womb of the Universe, the void that creates. The Valley (*gǔ*) is hollow, empty, low-lying: the space necessary for life to enter. The character *xuán* (玄) carries stellar meaning—the dark thread connecting what can be seen to what cannot, the black-red color of the northern sky where stars emerge from apparent void.

Daoist tradition located the cosmic correlate of the Mysterious Female at the celestial pole, the still point around which all stars revolve. The Pole Star was called the Great One (*Tài Yī*)—the unmoving center governing by stillness, the void palace from which celestial order emanates. The body mirrors these structures: the *dāntián* corresponds to the celestial pole; the meridians correspond to the Heavenly River. When the practitioner settles into genuine stillness, interior space opens to its cosmic correspondence. The microcosm aligns with the macrocosm. The gate appears.

The Gate is the point of conjunction—not opposition but union, the portal through which the unmanifested becomes manifest. In ordinary waking consciousness, *Yang* and *Yin* are differentiated. The Gate opens when this differentiation softens, when polarity relaxes toward the unity from which it emerged.

Sleep naturally moves in this direction. Consciousness releases its daytime grip. The practitioner of *Shuì Gōng* cooperates with this dissolution, maintaining interior awareness even as structures of waking identity release. This is not a battle. It is a return.

## Practical Approaches to the Gate

The Gate reveals itself through conditions, not seeking. You cannot storm it. You prepare. It opens.

These are not sequential steps but concurrent conditions. Each supports the others. Any single point can serve as an entry point.

### *The Valley Breath*

The Spirit of the Valley is empty, receptive, low-lying—receiving what flows down without grasping. Cultivate this in the breath. Do not breathe actively. Allow the breath to be breathed. Receive the inhale as the valley receives rain. Release the exhale as the valley releases mist. Let the breath settle lower and lower until it pools in the belly. The pooling creates the valley. The valley creates conditions for the Gate.

### *The Union of Fire and Water*

In the post-heaven arrangement, Fire rises and Water sinks. Heart-awareness ascends; Kidney-vitality descends. This is ordinary life: the mind floats upward into thinking while the body's vitality settles downward and stagnates. The practice reverses this drift. Let awareness sink from head toward belly. Let vitality rise from the lower back toward the heart. Where they meet—neither high nor low, neither front nor back—the Gate manifests.

### *The Cessation of the Acquired Mind*

The post-heaven mind generates content ceaselessly: memories, plans, evaluations, fantasies. This activity maintains the separation that keeps the Gate closed. When this mind settles completely, the pre-heaven mind reveals itself—original, unconditioned awareness. The Gate is not a door in space. It is a threshold in mind.

### *The Return of the Senses*

Ordinarily, the senses project outward—eyes capturing objects, ears capturing sounds, attention captured by phenomena. The reversal withdraws this projection. Eyes close or soften inward. Ears release their grip on sound. Touch withdraws from the skin surface toward the interior. This withdrawal creates the interiorization necessary for the Gate to appear.

### *The Softening of Identity*

The sense of separate self—bounded, defended, distinct—maintains the post-heaven condition. The Gate opens when this sense softens. Not through effort to dissolve the self, which only reinforces it, but through relaxation of the vigilance maintaining it. Sleep naturally softens identity. *Shuì Gōng* cooperates consciously. The Sleeping Immortal did not annihilate himself. He floated on mist and clouds.

## The Cultivation Sequence

The preceding practices can be done seated. What follows is the full reclining sequence, creating conditions for the Gate to reveal itself through sleep.

### *Preparation*

Before lying down, settle the energy accumulated in the head during the day. Modern life concentrates vitality in the upper body while depleting the lower. Draw energy downward. Ground. Settle.

Stand quietly, attention on the soles of the feet. Massage the feet, particularly Kidney-1, Bubbling Spring (*Yǒng Quán*). When heaviness and warmth fill the lower body, proceed.

## *The Reclining Posture*

Lie on the right side. Legs slightly bent. One hand under cheek or chin, the other resting on the thigh. This is the Sleeping Lion position—found in both Daoist and Buddhist traditions. Lying on the right slightly compresses the right nostril, calming mental activity.

Comfort matters. Discomfort generates agitation. The surface should be firm; too-soft beds allow the body to sink into positions obstructing energy flow.

## *The Physical Seals*

Several arrangements seal the body's energy. Tongue touches the roof of the mouth just behind the front teeth, completing a circuit between the two main channels. Eyes close or remain half-closed with soft downward orientation. Mouth gently closed. Anal sphincter is lightly contracted. These closures prevent leakage from the lower gates while the upper gates soften into receptivity.

## *The Breath Transition*

This stage distinguishes *Shuì Gōng* from ordinary falling asleep. Instead of allowing consciousness to dissolve into unconsciousness, maintain interior awareness while the breath undergoes transition.

Normal breathing: obvious movement of air through the nose. As you settle, breathing naturally softens. Slower. Finer. Less perceptible. The pause between breaths lengthens. Eventually, the sense of breathing relocates. Instead of air moving through the nostrils, there is a subtle pulsation in the lower belly. Daoist texts call this Embryonic Breathing (*Tàixī*): the state of a fetus in the womb, sustained without independent respiration.

This transition cannot be forced. Attempting to manipulate the breath creates exactly the tension preventing it. Observe. Allow.

Over weeks and months, the transition occurs earlier, more reliably. The breath becomes mist.

### *Genuine Sleep*

Beyond the breath transition lies genuine sleep (*zhēn shuì*). The body is profoundly still—hibernation more than rest. Dreams either do not arise or arise without capturing attention. Awareness is present but objectless. It rests in its own nature, luminous and empty.

This is what Chen Tuan meant: fundamentally without sleep, yet floating on mist and clouds. Not unconsciousness but radiant stillness. Not absence but presence without content. The practitioner who tastes this state—even briefly—understands why the sage remained on Mount Hua.

This state cannot be achieved through effort. It can only be allowed. The preceding stages create conditions. The Gate opens of itself or does not. The practitioner's task is preparation and patience. The Sleeping Immortal waited. So do we.

## Practical Matters

### *Gradual Approach*

The full practice represents mature development. Beginners start simply: the reclining posture, the physical seals, and natural breathing. The body learns the position; the mind learns to settle while lying down without immediately falling into ordinary unconsciousness. Over weeks and months, the breath naturally softens. Observe without manipulating; allow without grasping.

### *Regularity Over Intensity*

Brief daily practice establishes the pattern more effectively than occasional extended sessions. Using *Shuì Gōng* as the method of falling asleep each night provides a consistent opportunity. Even maintaining awareness through only the first few minutes before falling into ordinary sleep—those minutes accumulate. Each night, another approach to the Gate.

### *Environment*

The sleeping space should be dark, quiet, and slightly cool. Heat agitates; cold contracts. The surface should be firm enough to maintain posture. Traditional recommendations include sleeping with the head oriented to the east or north.

### *Diet and Evening Activity*

Heavy food before sleep obstructs settling. The final meal should be light, taken several hours before practice. Stimulants agitate; intoxicants dull. Mental activity before sleep generates residual momentum. The evening hours serve practice best when devoted to calming engagement.

## Markers of Progress

How do you know the practice is working? Not by dramatic experiences but by subtle shifts in the quality of sleep and waking.

### *Quality of Waking*

The most reliable marker is how you wake. Ordinary sleep produces gradual waking, residual grogginess, and the reluctant return. Genuine sleep produces instant, complete waking—clear mind, stable energy, no lag. The practitioner opens their eyes, already present. This clarity reflects the state achieved during sleep. Contact with the source—even briefly—leaves an imprint.

### *Restoration Ratio*

Genuine sleep restores more efficiently than ordinary sleep. Practitioners consistently report needing less sleep while feeling more rested. Ordinary sleep dissipates energy through dream-generation and restless movement. Genuine sleep consolidates. The body receives profound rest while the energetic system gains ground.

### *Dream Patterns*

As practice matures, dream patterns shift. Early stages may produce more vivid dreams as settled energy stirs dormant material—clearing, not regression. Later stages produce either dreamlessness or lucid presence within whatever arises. Dreams may occur but do not capture attention; they are witnessed without identification. Eventually, the distinction matters less. Both dreamlessness and lucid presence are modes of awareness resting in their own nature.

### *Daytime Effects*

Practice during sleep affects waking life. Increased equanimity. Reduced emotional reactivity. Clearer thinking. More stable energy throughout the day. The same settling that allows genuine sleep produces settling in waking consciousness. The Daoist literature describes this as a gradual return to simplicity—not simplification that loses complexity, but a prior simplicity that precedes complexity without excluding it.

## An Astrological Contribution

Classical astrology assigns the twelfth house to sleep, dissolution, and hidden matters. What follows extends this assignment into practical technology for *Shuì Gōng*. The term ruler analysis—using the bound lord of the twelfth cusp as threshold significator—is original to this work. Traditional sources do not apply the term rulership to sleep cultivation; the synthesis emerges from clinical practice, not textual transmission.

## The Twelfth House Cusp

The twelfth house governs sleep, dissolution, and hidden matters. Traditional astrology associates it with imprisonment, illness, secret enemies—but these share a common thread: the twelfth is where structures of waking identity weaken, where the conscious ego loses control, where something other operates. For sleep cultivation, this house describes the threshold between waking consciousness and whatever lies beyond.

## *Finding the Threshold Ruler*

Identify the degree of your twelfth house cusp. Then find which planet rules the term (or bound) of that degree. Each sign divides into five unequal segments, each ruled by a different planet. This term ruler is the significator of your sleep threshold—the planetary force governing passage from waking into deeper states.

## *Planets Residing in the Twelfth*

Planets in the twelfth house color the sleep experience directly. They are present at the threshold, active in the territory of dissolution.

*Sun in the twelfth.* Identity enters the hidden realm. The ego releases its grip readily—beneficial for dissolution, challenging for maintaining awareness. Dreams may feature authorities or guides. The task: dissolve without disappearing, release identity while retaining the witness thread.

*Moon in the twelfth.* The emotional body is attuned to the hidden. Dreams are vivid, richly textured, easily remembered. The threshold opens naturally. The challenge: moving beyond dream content into dreamless awareness. The Moon loves images; stillness beneath the play requires cultivation.

*Mercury in the twelfth.* The mind operates behind the scenes—restless, subtle, quick. Racing thoughts at the threshold, or unusual access to subtle perception. The challenge: quieting the acquired mind enough to receive what it seeks. Mercury must learn that some transmissions require silence.

*Venus in the twelfth.* Hidden pleasures, secret longings. Sleep becomes seductive—the practitioner enjoys dissolution too much to maintain awareness through it. The gate opens through relaxation and beauty. Yet attachment to the pleasure of dissolving is still attachment.

*Mars in the twelfth.* Restlessness at the threshold. Anger or fear surfacing as consciousness dissolves. The practitioner may fight sleep or wake repeatedly. Yet Mars provides energy others lack—the capacity to push through obstacles. True strength includes the strength to yield.

*Jupiter in the twelfth.* Natural capacity for the work. The *hún* is comfortable in hidden realms. Dreams are large, meaningful, and sometimes prophetic. The danger is spiritual inflation—mistaking vivid inner experience for attainment. Humility balances the gift.

*Saturn in the twelfth.* The threshold feels heavy, forbidding. Fear of dissolution, nameless dread surfacing as consciousness releases. Yet Saturn builds what others cannot: endurance. The practitioner who persists develops profound stability in deeper states.

*Rahu in the twelfth.* The North Node disrupts the threshold. Sleep may be irregular, punctuated by astral disturbances. The boundary between sleeping and waking blurs. Yet Rahu indicates strong past-life momentum toward spiritual practice. The challenge: distinguishing genuine subtle perception from Rahu's gift for illusion.

*Ketu in the twelfth.* The South Node finds its natural home. *Ketu* is the *mokṣa kāraka*—significator of liberation—, and the twelfth is liberation's domain. Dissolution comes naturally, sometimes too naturally. Of all placements, Ketu in the twelfth house most favors *Shuì Gōng*. The gate stands already ajar.

## Assessing the Term Ruler

*Well-dignified* (domicile, exaltation, strong triplicity): The gate opens readily. Natural capacity for the transition. Practice proceeds smoothly.

*Peregrine* (holding no essential dignity): The gate is neutral. Progress depends on consistent practice rather than innate facility.

*Debilitated* (detriment or fall): Obstacles at the threshold. The practitioner may approach the gate but find it closed, or cross briefly but be unable to sustain the state.

*Afflicted by malefics* (Saturn or Mars in hard aspect): Specific obstacles appear. Saturn: heaviness, fear. Mars: restlessness, heat, intrusive thoughts.

### *Working with the Significator*

*Sun-ruled threshold:* Diminish self-reference before sleep. The Organ Gaze works particularly well—warmth without self-assertion.

*Moon-ruled threshold:* Generally favorable. If afflicted, practice emotional clearing before sleep.

*Mercury-ruled threshold:* Avoid mental work before practice. The breath practices give the mind something to attend to.

*Venus-ruled threshold:* Practice non-attachment to the pleasantness of settling.

*Mars-ruled threshold:* Cool the system before practice. Avoid stimulants, intense exercise, heated conversations.

*Jupiter-ruled threshold:* Practice restraint in the evening. Avoid stimulation that Jupiter amplifies.

*Saturn-ruled threshold:* Practice earlier when some *Yang* vitality remains. Cultivate felt sense of safety.

## Summing this Chapter

The practice of *Shuì Gōng* is a return—a reversal of the current that ordinarily carries the human spirit toward depletion. By retracing the path from the Ten Thousand Things back to the Five Agents, and from the Five Agents back to the Great Pole, the practitioner seeks the unmoving center.

The Gate of the Mysterious Female is not a destination to be reached but a threshold to be allowed. It is the "root of Heaven and Earth," the dark thread connecting manifest reality to the Pre-Celestial source. When the practitioner settles into the Sleeping Lion posture, completes the physical seals, and transitions from atmospheric breathing to Embryonic Breath, they are not merely resting. They are participating in cosmic alignment.

Your natal chart provides the map for this crossing. By identifying your term ruler and understanding the planetary guests residing in your house of dissolution, you transform a period of unconsciousness into a laboratory of the spirit.

The goal of Daoist Sleep Cultivation is to wake before you open your eyes. Return from the depths carrying the Joy of the Sun in your marrow. What the Sleeping Immortal discovered on Mount Hua remains available: the gate stands open every night.

We cross now into territory where interpretation itself transforms. The Tibetan tradition developed something no other system attempted: technology for practicing *within* the dream. The celestial framework remains—elements, vital forces, birth calculations—but the aim shifts from reading the dream to using it. The nightly journey becomes a rehearsal for the bardo encountered at death.

# Note

Liu Ming (1947–2016), born Charles Belyea, studied in Taiwan for over a decade before founding Da Yuan Circle in Oakland, California, where he transmitted Daoist arts until his death. He organized dream work into three progressive layers—Healing, Divination, and Path—the last of which forms the subject of this chapter.

# Sources

Bisio, Tom. *Daoist Sleeping Meditation: Chen Tuan's Sleeping Gong*. Denver: Outskirts Press, 2021.

Ekirch, A. Roger. *At Day's Close: Night in Times Past*. New York: W.W. Norton, 2005.

Hausen, Johan, and Aaron Tsaur. *The Arts of Daoism*. Auckland: Purple Cloud Press, 2021.

Kohn, Livia. *Internal Alchemy: Self, Society, and the Quest for Immortality*. Cambridge, MA: Three Pines Press, 2009.

———. *Sitting in Oblivion: The Heart of Daoist Meditation*. Cambridge, MA: Three Pines Press, 2010.

———. *Taoist Meditation and Longevity Techniques*. Ann Arbor: Center for Chinese Studies, University of Michigan, 1989.

Komjathy, Louis. *Traces of a Daoist Immortal: Chén Tuán of the Western Marchmount*. Leiden: Brill, 2024.

Laozi. *Dàodé Jīng*. Translations consulted: D.C. Lau (Penguin, 1963); Victor Mair (Bantam, 1990); Red Pine (Copper Canyon, 2009).

Liu Ming. Oral teachings, Da Yuan Circle, Oakland, California, 1990s–2016.

Liu Yiming. *Cultivating the Tao: Taoism and Internal Alchemy*. Translated by Fabrizio Pregadio. Mountain View: Golden Elixir Press, 2013.

Pregadio, Fabrizio. *The Seal of the Unity of the Three: A Study and Translation of the Cantong qi*. Mountain View: Golden Elixir Press, 2011.

Robinet, Isabelle. *Taoist Meditation: The Mao-Shan Tradition of Great Purity*. Translated by Julian Pas and Norman Girardot. Albany: SUNY Press, 1993.

Zhang Jingyue. *Lèi Jīng* (Classic of Categories), 1624. Dream interpretation chapters excerpted in Hausen and Tsaur (2021).

Zhou Lüjing. *Chì Fèng Suǐ* (The Marrow of the Red Phoenix), 1578. Excerpts in Bisio (2021).

## Chapter Nine

# Bön Dream Yoga: The Tibetan Path

*If we cannot carry our practice into sleep, if we lose ourselves every night, what chance do we have to be aware when death comes?*

*—Tenzin Wangyal Rinpoche*

Bön sits beyond the external-internal spectrum, not along it. Dreams are neither messages to interpret nor symptoms to diagnose. The dream becomes a practice space—a field for transformation. The practitioner enters actively, rehearsing for the *bardo* states encountered at death.

## The Zhang Zhung Inheritance

Zhang Zhung developed a complete system: Yungdrung Bön, the Eternal Bön. Among its treasures is a technology for working with consciousness during sleep.

Before Buddhism reached Tibet, this kingdom flourished around Mount Kailash—a distinct nation, its own language and script, capital at Khyunglung, the Silver Palace of Garuda. Tibet annexed Zhang Zhung in the 8th century, assassinating King Ligmincha. The synthesis absorbed Bön worldview, medicine, and ritual into Buddhist teaching. This heritage survives in the Mother Tantra (*Ma Gyud*) cycles, which emphasize completion-stage practice and direct realization of the mind's nature through sleep.

Bön traces its teachings to Tönpa Shenrap Miwoche, said to have lived eighteen thousand years ago in the mythical Olmo Lungring. Historical figure or archetypal source, Shenrap transmitted the Way of the Shen of Prediction (*phywa gshen theg pa*)—astrology, divination, medicine, and what became dream yoga. Tradition holds that Shenrap transformed Bön from its earlier phase of animistic ritual and animal sacrifice into Yungdrung Bön, replacing blood offerings with symbolic *tormas* of barley flour and butter.

This historical shift parallels dream yoga's internal movement: from passive reception to active transformation. Untamed energies of the unconscious redirect toward enlightenment.

This chapter examines Bön dream yoga within its celestial framework: five elements, nine *mewa*, eight *parkha*, four vital forces, and six realms.

# The Tibetan Celestial Framework

Tibetan astrology synthesizes Bön, Chinese, and Indian systems. The result differs from all sources. Internal coherence remains. For dream yoga, this framework provides timing, diagnosis, and orientation within the cycles governing human experience.

## *The Five Elements*

Wood, Fire, Earth, Metal, Water. Same elements as Chinese astrology, but with a distinctive Bön interpretation. Each governs specific qualities and correlates with the vital forces that dream practice addresses.

*Table 9.1. The Five Elements and Vital Forces*

| Element | Quality | Vital Force | Dream Sign | Season |
|---|---|---|---|---|
| Wood | Growth, expansion | *Lungta* | Trees, spring imagery, growth | Spring |
| Fire | Transformation, clarity | *Wangthang* | Light, burning, illumination | Summer |
| Earth | Stability, nourishment | *Lus* | Ground, buildings, solidity | Transitions |
| Metal | Contraction, boundaries | *Srog* | Weapons, cutting, harvesting | Autumn |
| Water | Flowing, depth | *La* | Rivers, oceans, immersion | Winter |

Elements cycle through years, months, days. Dream yoga during Fire periods differs from practice during Water periods—not in technique but in what arises and what obstacles appear. The dreaming mind is not separate from biological and environmental conditions. A practitioner dreaming of floods during a Water period encounters elemental excess requiring balance through breathwork or visualization. Elemental medicine treats the dream as a real-time monitor of the subtle body's alignment with the cosmos.

## The Four Vital Forces

Bön astrology identifies four forces governing human flourishing. Dreams reveal their state; practice strengthens them.

*Srog* is life force—vital energy sustaining existence. When weak, dreams turn toward death, dissolution, endings. Practice during *srog* weakness focuses on stabilization, not expansion.

*Lus* governs the body and health. Dreams of illness, injury, bodily distortion indicate *lus* disturbance. The astrologer examines current conditions and advises whether the practice should address physical grounding.

*Wangthang* relates to power, capacity, and accomplishment. Dreams of success or failure, wealth or poverty, recognition or humiliation reflect *wangthang* condition. Western astrology might call this fortune or dignity.

*Lungta*—wind horse—is distinctively Tibetan. Forward momentum, confidence, auspicious movement. The image: a horse carrying the wish-fulfilling jewel across the sky. Dreams of flying, riding, and swift travel indicate strong *lungta*. Dreams of being stuck, weighted down, and unable to move indicate depletion. Raising prayer flags strengthens *lungta*; dream yoga offers internal methods.

## The Nine Mewa

The nine *mewa* form a magic square cycling through years, months, days. Each has specific qualities, elemental ties, and practice implications. The system derives from Chinese sources but receives distinctive Bön elaboration—particularly regarding *bardo* experience.

*Table 9.2. The Nine Mewa and Bardo Implications*

| Mewa | Color | Element | Quality | Bardo Implication |
|---|---|---|---|---|
| 1 | White | Iron | Clarity, beginnings | Clear light may dawn easily |
| 2 | Black | Water | Depth, obstacles | Risk of confusion |
| 3 | Blue | Water | Communication, movement | May encounter guides |
| 4 | Green | Wood | Growth, healing | Favorable rebirth |
| 5 | Yellow | Earth | Center, power | Strong presence; can go either way |
| 6 | White | Iron | Completion, protection | Protection from lower realms |
| 7 | Red | Fire | Passion, intensity | Risk of wrathful visions |
| 8 | White | Iron | Stillness, contemplation | Favorable for recognition |
| 9 | Red | Fire | Culmination, transformation | Intensity at transition |

Sometimes called the Magic Square of Saturn—connection to time, karma, cyclic structures. Birth *mewa* indicates innate tendencies; current *mewa* indicates present conditions. Those born under *mewa* 2 may experience more obstacle dreams, requiring intensive foundational work to achieve lucidity; those under 1 or 8 may find clarity arising easily.

## *The Eight Parkha*

Eight trigrams from Chinese *ba gua*, with Tibetan interpretation. Each consists of three lines—broken or unbroken—representing configurations of elemental force. The *parkha* governs directions, family relationships, spatial orientation, including the orientation of the sleeping body.

Traditional instruction specifies sleeping positions based on *parkha* calculation. Birth *parkha* indicates favorable and unfavorable directions. Sleeping with the head toward an unfavorable direction may disturb dreams or obstruct practice. The lion's posture (*senge gyalwey neypa*)—right side, right hand under cheek—is standard. Directional orientation depends on individual calculation.

Consciousness is not placeless during sleep. The mind remains tethered to a body that is itself a node within a larger celestial grid. Aligning the physical body with *parkha* and *mewa* optimizes the flow of wisdom-*prāṇa* through the central channel, increasing the likelihood that dreams of clarity emerge over ordinary *saṃsāric* dreams.

## The Six Realms and Dream Consciousness

Tibetan cosmology maps existence into six realms of rebirth—literal destinations after death, psychological states accessible nightly. Sleep opens onto these territories. Dream content reveals which realm consciousness has entered.

The god realm (*lha*) produces dreams of bliss, ease, floating, and golden light. Pleasant—but spiritually dangerous. The dreamer absorbed in divine pleasure cultivates complacency; no urgency drives transformation. These dreams seduce.

The jealous god realm (*lha ma yin*) generates dreams of competition, struggle, and warfare. The dreamer fights, schemes, and measures against rivals. Ambition without satisfaction. Victory leads only to the next battle.

The human realm (*mi*) yields mixed dreams—pleasure and pain, gain and loss, choice and consequence. The dreamer navigates, decides, and acts. Of all realms, human birth offers optimal conditions for awakening: enough suffering to motivate practice, enough ease to sustain it.

The animal realm (*dud 'gro*) manifests as instinctual dreams—pursuit, flight, feeding, mating. Confusion dominates. The dreamer reacts without reflection, driven by survival imperatives, unable to step back and observe.

The hungry ghost realm (*yi dvags*) fills dreams with craving and lack. Food that cannot be eaten. Water that cannot be drunk. Endless seeking, no satisfaction. The dreamer wakes exhausted, still wanting.

The hell realm (*dmyal ba*) is nightmare territory—suffering, entrapment, torment. Heat or cold. Pursuit by hostile forces. The dreamer cannot escape, cannot wake, endures.

## *Celestial Correlations*

The twelve houses divide into six axes, each a polarity. Each polarity maps onto a realm:

*Table 9.3. House Axes and the Six Realms*

| Axis | Houses | Realm | Signature |
|---|---|---|---|
| 1–7 | Self–Other | *Human (mi)* | Relationship, choice, negotiation |
| 2–8 | Resource–Transformation | *Hungry Ghost (yi dvags)* | Accumulation, loss, craving |
| 3–9 | Knowledge–Wisdom | *Jealous God (lha ma yin)* | Mental competition, doctrinal struggle |
| 4–10 | Root–Manifestation | *Animal (dud 'gro)* | Security instinct, territorial drive |
| 5–11 | Creation–Community | *God (lha)* | Pleasure, abundance, ease |
| 6–12 | Service–Dissolution | *Hell (dmyal ba)* | Suffering, confinement, expiation |

The axis containing the natal Moon indicates the realm of consciousness that defaults toward in sleep. Moon in the second or eighth: hungry ghost territory—dreams of lack, craving, resource anxiety. Moon in the sixth or twelfth: hell realm proximity—dreams of illness, imprisonment, dissolution. Moon on the 5–11 axis: god realm pull—pleasant dreams offering no traction for transformation.

Transits activate realm-signatures. Saturn crossing the 2–8 axis intensifies hungry ghost themes; the dreamer reports scarcity, theft, and losing what was possessed. Mars transiting 6–12 ignites hell realm material—nightmares, entrapment, bodily suffering. Jupiter crossing 5–11 opens god realm territory—dreams so pleasant the dreamer resists waking.

## *Emotional Signatures*

Each realm carries a characteristic emotional tone that manifests in both dream content and waking disposition:

*Table 9.4. Realms, Emotions, and Vital Force Correlations*

| Realm | Emotion | Weakened Force | Dream Signs | Remedial Approach |
|---|---|---|---|---|
| Hell | Anger | *Srog* | Death, pursuit, torment | Life-force mantras; protective practice |
| Hungry Ghost | Greed | *Lungta* | Lack, craving, inability to consume | Raise prayer flags; generosity practice |
| Animal | Ignorance | *Lus* | Instinct, confusion, pursuit/flight | Physical grounding; medical attention |
| Human | Jealousy | *Wangthang* | Competition, comparison, measuring | Empowerment rituals; accomplish goals |
| Jealous God | Pride | *Wangthang* | Warfare, struggle, ambition | Humility practice; offering victory |
| God | Lethargic pleasure | *Lungta* | Bliss, floating, ease | Renunciation; generate urgency |

The practitioner uses recurring dream themes as diagnostic data. Persistent competition dreams indicate jealous god realm habitation. Persistent scarcity dreams indicate hungry ghost territory. The natal chart shows predisposition; transits show activation; dream content confirms.

## *Diagnostic Application*

Recurring dreams reveal habitual tendencies. A patient whose dreams consistently feature competition and struggle drifts toward the jealous god realm—and likely carries that orientation into waking life. One whose dreams circle endlessly around what cannot be obtained inhabits hungry ghost territory.

This is not metaphor. The realms name actual configurations of mind-energy. The dreamer experiencing hell-realm nightmare genuinely suffers; the dreamer floating in god-realm bliss genuinely misses the opportunity suffering provides.

A patient with Moon in the eighth, Pluto now conjunct natal Moon, reports recurring dreams of burial, loss, watching loved ones die. Hell realm has opened—cosmically triggered, experientially real. Treatment addresses both levels: the transit (timing, duration, meaning) and the realm (recognition practice, compassion cultivation).

### *Transformational Practice*

Recognition is the first intervention. The dreamer trained to identify realm-signatures can, upon recognizing where they are, shift the dream's trajectory. Bön *milam* teaches specific techniques: in the jealous god realm, cease fighting and offer victory to the opponent; in the hungry ghost realm, visualize giving away what is craved; in the hell realm, recognize tormentors as projections and offer compassion.

Seed syllables purify realm-karma at its root. The six syllables of the Mani mantra—OM MA NI PAD ME HUNG—each address one realm. Sounding the appropriate syllable within the dream clears the karmic seed before it manifests in waking life.

The six realms practice bridges dream yoga and *bardo* preparation. At death, consciousness moves through intermediate states where the same realms appear—more vividly, with higher stakes. The dreamer who has spent years recognizing realms in sleep carries that recognition into dying. What was practice becomes navigation. The technology tested nightly proves itself when needed most.

## The Structure of Practice

Bön dream yoga moves from daytime preparation through nocturnal practice to morning integration.

## *Three Types of Dream Experience*

Bön identifies three types of dream experience.

Ordinary *saṃsāric* dreams arise from personal karmic traces (*bak-chak*). The mind recycles daily events, anxieties, and unfulfilled desires. Strong subject-object dichotomy. Usually non-lucid. The dreamer is passive, swept by karmic *prāṇa*.

Dreams of clarity occur when mind and *prāṇa* are balanced and the practitioner maintains non-personal presence. Unlike *saṃsāric* dreams, which project individual ego, dreams of clarity present knowledge arising from transpersonal consciousness. Prophetic insights, messages from teachers, encounters with deities.

Clear light dreams represent the highest level. Non-dual awareness (*rigpa*) where subject-object dichotomy dissolves. No imagery—only luminous, empty awareness. The goal: maintain awareness even when dream content is absent, mirroring the realization of the mind's nature in waking life.

The transition from *saṃsāric* dreams to dreams of clarity marks a critical milestone. The practitioner no longer reads psychological residue but accesses wisdom-*prāṇa*, connecting the individual to the larger enlightened field.

## *Four Daytime Foundations*

Dream yoga begins during the day. Four foundations.

*Changing karmic traces:* Throughout the day, cultivate awareness that experience is dreamlike—insubstantial, impermanent, empty. Not philosophy, but felt shift. When waking life is recognized as dreamlike, the boundary between waking and sleeping becomes permeable. Karmic traces that normally produce solid-seeming experience begin loosening.

*Removing grasping and aversion:* Strong attachment and aversion produce heavy traces, dense dreams. Meet all experiences—pleasant, unpleasant, neutral—with equanimity. Not emotional flatness but spacious awareness containing strong feelings without capture.

*Strengthening intention:* Multiple times daily, generate a clear intention to recognize the dream state. Not mere wish but *saṅkalpa*—vow penetrating to the deepest mind. "Tonight I will recognize the dream. I will know I am dreaming." Repetition plants intention, so it activates during sleep.

*Cultivating memory:* Review dreams on waking. Maintain enthusiasm for practice. Dream recall strengthens with attention; neglected dreams fade. Keep a journal. Discuss dreams with teachers or fellow practitioners.

Lucidity is not a switch flipped at night but a state cultivated twenty-four hours a day. If the daytime mind is scattered or reactive, the nighttime mind follows.

## *Four Nighttime Phases*

As sleep approaches, there are four phases of practice—each with a chakra, a seed syllable, and a quality of awareness. Not rigidly sequential. Experience teaches which phase serves in any moment.

*Throat chakra (A):* Visualize a luminous red Tibetan A at the throat. The primordial sound, basis of manifestation. Quality: peaceful presence—relaxed awareness, not effort. Fall asleep with attention gently at the throat, A glowing softly. Supports the transition from waking to sleep, maintains continuity through hypnagogia.

*Brow chakra (OM):* If awareness is maintained or regained during the night, shift focus to the third eye. White OM. Quality: clarity—seeing the dream clearly, recognizing its nature, directing attention within it. Dreams become vivid, detailed, and easier to remember. The OM illuminates the dreamscape, making images stable, necessary for maintaining recognition.

*Heart chakra (HUNG):* Blue HUNG at the heart center. Deepest practice. Beyond recognizing dreams—resting in the nature of mind itself. *Rigpa,* pure awareness, equally present in waking, dreaming, and deep sleep. Dreams may continue, but are recognized as play of awareness, not something happening to a separate self.

*Secret chakra:* The fourth phase works with the generative center. Typically taught through direct transmission. A black *thigle* (sphere of light) visualized at this center develops fearlessness—courage to face the radical dissolution of elements occurring in deep sleep and death.

These phases are not strictly sequential but represent energetic keys. If the dream is hazy, focus on the brow; if frightening, focus on the secret chakra; if the goal is pure awareness, focus on the heart.

### *The Role of the Dakini Salgye Du Dalma*

Within the Mother Tantra tradition, a specific guardian deity oversees practice: the *ḍākinī* Salgye Du Dalma ("She Who Clarifies Beyond Conception"). She is the luminosity hidden within the darkness of normal sleep. Practitioners develop a relationship with her essence during the day, visualizing her as a pure white, luminous body of light.

Before sleep, imagine dissolving into her, mixing essence until practitioner and *ḍākinī* are one. She reminds the practitioner to remain in the presence and cut through ignorance. Not an external goddess but a representation of the practitioner's own deepest nature—inherently clear and luminous.

## Working with Dream Content

Once lucidity is established—knowing, within the dream, that dreaming is occurring—specific practices transform the dream from experience to training.

*Transformation:* Change dream content deliberately. Fire becomes water; enemies become friends; small becomes large. Not escapism but training in malleability. If dream fire can become water through intention, the practitioner begins understanding: phenomena arise through conditions; mind influences them.

*Multiplication:* One flower becomes a thousand. One body becomes many. Loosens attachment to singularity, fixed identity.

*Emanation:* Emanate as different forms—animals, elements, deities. Develops capacity for multiple perspectives. Prepares for *bardo* experiences where form is fluid, and identity is no longer bound to the human body.

*Journey:* Travel within dreams to pure lands—dimensions associated with enlightened beings. Deepen connection with enlightened qualities, receive direct teachings from lineage masters. Whether actual locations, states of consciousness, or symbolic encounters, such journeys deepen connection with awakened qualities.

## Dream Yoga as Bardo Preparation

The Tibetan tradition identifies multiple *bardo* states—transitions occurring not only at death but throughout life. Dream *bardo* (*milam bardo*) is one of six. Mastery here prepares for the others, particularly *chikhai bardo* (moment of death) and *chönyid bardo* (luminous visions after death).

The connection is not an analogy. According to Bön teaching, the same processes occur in falling asleep as in dying: dissolution of elements, withdrawal from senses, arising of visionary experience, and emergence of clear light. One who maintains awareness through sleep transition has trained for death transition. One who recognizes dreams as dreams has trained for recognizing *bardo* visions as visions—not solid reality requiring reactive response.

The *mewa* system explicitly addresses this. Each *mewa* carries implications for *bardo* experience—whether clarity arises easily or confusion predominates, whether guides appear or wrathful visions threaten. Dream yoga allows working with these tendencies before death. Strengthen the favorable, purify the obstacles.

### *The Dissolution Sequence*

As the body falls asleep—and as it dies—elements dissolve in sequence. Each dissolution produces signs that the trained practitioner recognizes.

*Table 9.5. The Dissolution Sequence*

| Dissolution | Physical Sign | Inner Sign | Dream Correlation |
|---|---|---|---|
| Earth → Water | Body heavy, sinking | Mirage appearance | Hypnagogic heaviness |
| Water → Fire | Fluids dry | Smoke appearance | Diffuse imagery |
| Fire → Wind | Heat withdraws | Sparks, fireflies | Flashing lights |
| Wind → Consciousness | Breath ceases | Steady flame | Stable dream imagery forms |
| White appearance | (subtle level) | White light, moonlight | Bright, spacious dreams |
| Red increase | (subtle level) | Red light, sunset | Warm, vivid dreams |
| Black near-attainment | (subtle level) | Darkness, void | Gap before REM |
| Clear light | (very subtle) | Luminous emptiness | Recognition of awareness |

The hypnagogic period—liminal zone between waking and sleep—becomes training ground for the *bardo*. Flashing lights, falling sensation, dissolving body-sense: meet with awareness rather than unconsciousness. The practitioner who remains present through black near-attainment into clear light has accomplished something that will serve at death.

# Celestial Timing

Bön astrology provides specific guidance: when to undertake practice, what to expect during different periods. Work with cycles of *mewa*, *parkha*, and elements to optimize conditions.

## *Favorable and Unfavorable Periods*

Certain *mewa* days support practice; others present obstacles. When current *mewa* matches birth *mewa*—*mewa gu-mik*, ninth-spot—a period of transition arises. Dreams may be unusually vivid or disturbing. Work with this intensity, or emphasize protection.

*Dur-mik* (death-spot) identifies periods of vulnerability based on birth sign and current *parkha*. The name sounds ominous, but these periods offer opportunity for deep practice. Conditions difficult for ordinary activity can support intensive retreat and dream work.

The lunar cycle governs practice. Waxing moon supports expansion—practices aimed at developing clarity and lucidity. Waning moon supports release—practices aimed at dissolving obstacles and purifying traces. The full moon is especially powerful. Lunar energy supports visionary experience; many practitioners report spontaneous lucidity.

## The Clear Light

Beyond lucid dreaming, beyond transformation, beyond *bardo* preparation: recognition of *ösel*, the clear light. Luminous nature of mind, present in waking, dreaming, and deep sleep—ordinarily obscured. Not a particular experience, but the ground of all experience. Awareness within which phenomena arise.

In ordinary sleep, clear light dawns briefly in transition from waking to dreaming—the moment of black near-attainment before dreams form. Most sleepers pass through unconsciously. Dream yoga trains recognition of this moment. Rest in clear light rather than grasping at dream content. With practice, clear light sustains longer. Eventually recognized not only in sleep but in waking life.

Here, dream yoga transcends interpretation. Earlier chapters read dreams for meaning—omens, diagnosis, prophecy. Bön uses dreams as a doorway to something beyond meaning: direct recognition of awareness itself. Neither requires interpretation nor produces interpretable content. The dream becomes support for awakening, not text to decode.

Yet even this ultimate aim connects to celestial framework. *Mewa* and *parkha* calculations identify conditions supporting or obstructing clear light recognition. Certain birth configurations indicate innate capacity; others indicate need for more preparation. The astrologer advises when conditions favor intensive clear light practice. Highest spiritual aims integrated with practical celestial timing.

## Clinical Parallels

Bön overlaps with modern lucid dreaming research. Stephen LaBerge's Mnemonic Induction of Lucid Dreams (MILD) parallels the Bön foundation of strengthening intention. Cognitive science recognizes that metacognitive awareness during sleep activates prefrontal and parietal regions associated with self-reflection and executive control.

A fundamental difference emerges: Western lucid dreaming often focuses on control for psychological healing or entertainment. Bön dream yoga uses control as a preliminary to releasing. The goal is not to become the god of the dream world but to use the dream's malleability to prove its emptiness. Once the mind is convinced of the dream's illusory nature, it can rest in clear light beyond imagery and control.

## The Tibetan Contribution

Bön dream yoga offers what no other tradition in this volume provides: systematic technology for transforming consciousness within the dream, integrated with celestial medicine. Where Mesopotamia reads divine message, where Chinese medicine reads organ-spirit feedback, where Vedic astrology validates prophetic content, Bön enters the dream as a practice field.

Elements, *mewa*, *parkha*, vital forces, six realms—celestial scaffolding for practice. Not working in isolation but in conscious relationship with cosmic cycles. Timing by *mewa* calculation. Body orientation by *parkha* direction. Vital force diagnosis through dream content. Realm recognition through house-axis awareness. *Bardo* preparation through nightly rehearsal.

## The Westward Turn

We have traveled eastward along the internalization spectrum—from the Mesopotamian temple where dreams arrived as a divine message, through the Egyptian threshold where constitution shaped reception, to the Indian timing protocols, Chinese organ-spirit diagnostics, and

Tibetan practice technology. Each tradition pushed the locus of dream experience further inward.

A parallel stream flows westward. While India and China developed internal cosmologies of the dreaming mind, the Hellenistic world accomplished something distinct: mathematical formalization of celestial influence, systematic correlation of planetary conditions with dream veracity, and protocols for determining whether a dream spoke truth or phantasm. This current—Greek philosophical cosmology through Persian synthesis to Arabic transmission to Latin codification—produced the technical apparatus Western medical astrology still employs.

Artemidorus distinguished non-predictive dreams (*enhypnia*), arising from bodily imbalance or daily anxiety, from predictive dreams (*oneiroi*), divinely sent or soul-derived. His method emphasized knowing the dreamer's background to determine veracity—paralleling Bön's vital forces as a baseline for interpretation.

Bonatti codified these principles into a systematic horary framework. His considerations for testing phantasm versus truth serve the same function as Bön foundational practices: clearing the noise of *saṃsāric* projection to reveal what is truly significant.

We turn west now to trace this other river.

## Sources

Chögyal Namkhai Norbu. *Dream Yoga and the Practice of Natural Light*. Edited by Michael Katz. Ithaca: Snow Lion, 1992.

Chögyal Namkhai Norbu. *The Crystal and the Way of Light*. Edited by John Shane. Ithaca: Snow Lion, 2000.

Cornu, Philippe. *Tibetan Astrology*. Translated by Hamish Gregor. Boston: Shambhala, 1997.

Henning, Edward. *Kālacakra and the Tibetan Calendar*. New York: Columbia University Press, 2007.

Holecek, Andrew. *Dream Yoga: Illuminating Your Life Through Lucid Dreaming*. Boulder: Sounds True, 2016.

Men-Tsee-Khang. *Tibetan Astronomy and Astrology: A Brief Introduction*. Dharamsala: Men-Tsee-Khang, 1995.

Mullin, Glenn H. *The Six Yogas of Naropa*. Ithaca: Snow Lion, 2005.

Tenzin Wangyal Rinpoche. *The Tibetan Yogas of Dream and Sleep*. Ithaca: Snow Lion, 1998.

Tenzin Wangyal Rinpoche. *Wonders of the Natural Mind*. Barrytown: Station Hill, 1993.

## Chapter Ten

# The Greek Synthesis

*πάντων μὲν θεὸς ἡγεμών*

*pantōn men theos hēgemōn*

*"God is the guide of all things."*

—Artemidorus, Oneirocritica I.2

On the external-internal spectrum, Greek synthesis stands midway. Artemidorus distinguishes *oneiros*—the prophetic dream that speaks from beyond—from *enhypnion*—the body talking to itself. Macrobius locates both within a Neoplatonic architecture of planetary descent. The Greeks preserved external possibility while systematizing criteria for internal causes. Divine message and bodily noise coexist. The interpreter's first task: tell them apart.

## The Reunion of Streams

The preceding chapters traced oneiromancy eastward—Mesopotamian divine visitation becoming Egyptian threshold-crossing becoming Indian temporal precision becoming Chinese organ-spirit diagnostics becoming Tibetan practice technology. Each tradition internalized the dream more fully. The journey reached its limit where interpretation dissolves into direct recognition.

We return now to the Mediterranean basin, where a parallel development unfolded. The Hellenistic period accomplished something unprecedented: the systematic integration of Babylonian zodiacal astrology, Egyptian decanal timing, and Greek philosophical cosmology into a unified framework for understanding celestial influence on human experience.

This synthesis matured between the second century BCE and the seventh century CE, reaching its most elaborate form under Sassanid Persian patronage, where works by Dorotheus of Sidon and Vettius Valens were translated into Pahlavi and integrated with Persian theological concerns. The resulting tradition treated the cosmos as a living architecture of meaning. Every soul was born into a pattern; dreams opened that pattern nightly—when the grip of waking loosened.

Three figures anchor the Greek contribution to oneiromancy: Artemidorus, who transformed dream interpretation into a systematic *technē*; Macrobius, who located dreams within the Neoplatonic cosmology of planetary spheres; and Asclepius—or rather, his temple cult—which institutionalized therapeutic dream incubation. Behind all three stands the astrological framework that provided celestial context for nocturnal experience.

# Artemidorus: The Technical Method

Artemidorus of Daldis composed his *Oneirocritica* (Interpretation of Dreams) around 200 CE—the only complete dream interpretation manual to survive from antiquity. Unlike the omen lists of Mesopotamia or the temple records of Egypt, Artemidorus offered a systematic method grounded in empirical observation. He had traveled extensively, collecting dreams and their outcomes, testing interpretive principles against actual fulfillment. His approach was a *technē*—craft, not gift. Learnable skill.

## *The Fundamental Distinction*

Artemidorus established a distinction that remains foundational. *Enhypnion* (within-sleep) processes daily residue—the thirsty person dreams of water, the anxious person dreams of their anxieties. These dreams vanish upon waking and carry no prophetic weight. They are mental housekeeping, the psyche digesting the day's impressions.

*Oneiros* (dream proper) is different. The word itself suggests disclosure—*eirein to on*, 'to reveal what is.' These dreams stir the soul and point toward future events. They arrive with a quality of communication, as if something wishes to be known. The *oneiros* demands interpretation; the *enhypnion* requires only recognition of its source.

This distinction parallels the Vedic separation of *bhāvika* (prophetic) dreams from the six other categories that reflect psychological processing or humoral disturbance. Both traditions recognized that most dreams carry no oracular weight—and that the interpreter's first task is classification.

## *Theorematic and Allegorical*

Within the category of significant dreams, Artemidorus distinguished *theorematikoi* (theorematic) from *allēgorikoi* (allegorical). A sailor dreams of a shipwreck; he then shipwrecks. This is theorematic—literal fulfillment. Most prophetic dreams, however, speak otherwise. They encode their meaning in metaphor, requiring skilled interpretation to decode.

The interpreter must know the dreamer. Artemidorus insisted on contextual assessment: occupation, health, age, social position, habits, and current circumstances. A single image signifies differently for different dreamers. Flying might indicate noble ambition for a person of high status, but predict instability for a commoner. The dream of losing teeth—a near-universal symbol—requires knowing whether the dreamer has dependents (teeth may signify family members) or debts (teeth may signify resources).

Body provided a substitution code. Head represents father; feet represent slaves; right hand represents son, brother, or friend; left hand represents wife, mother, or mistress. Physical injury in dreams translates to harm affecting the corresponding person in waking life. This somatic symbolism appears across cultures and anticipates later melothesia—the mapping of zodiacal signs and planets onto body parts.

### *Scope of Dreams*

Artemidorus classified dreams by scope. *Idioi* (personal) dreams affect the dreamer alone. *Demosioi* (public) dreams concern the city or community—the dreamer sees events that will affect many. *Kosmikoi* (cosmic) dreams signal universal events: eclipses, plagues, and the death of rulers. This classification acknowledges that dreams can operate at different scales of significance. The interpreter must assess not only what the dream means but how widely its meaning extends.

## Macrobius: The Neoplatonic Ladder

Ambrosius Theodosius Macrobius, writing around 400 CE, integrated dream theory with the Neoplatonic cosmology of planetary spheres in his *Commentary on the Dream of Scipio*. Where Artemidorus provided an empirical method, Macrobius provided a metaphysical framework. His five-fold taxonomy of dreams became the standard classification throughout the medieval period.

### *The Five Types*

*Somnium* (enigmatic dream): The symbolic dream requiring interpretation. It speaks in riddles and metaphors, concealing its meaning beneath surface imagery. Most significant dreams fall into this category. The interpreter's skill lies in penetrating the symbol to reach the signified.

*Visio* (prophetic vision): The dream that shows future events exactly as they will occur. No interpretation is needed—the dream is its own meaning. The sleeper sees tomorrow's shipwreck, tomorrow's visitor, tomorrow's news. These dreams are rare but unmistakable.

*Oraculum* (oracular dream): A divine figure, ancestor, or person of authority appears and gives direct instruction. The god speaks; the parent advises; the priest commands. The content requires not interpretation but obedience. This category preserves the ancient understanding of dreams as divine communication—the *dūta* (messenger) of Vedic tradition, the gods speaking through the sleeping threshold.

*Insomnium* (nightmare): The worthless dream caused by mental or physical distress.

*Macrobius* aligned this with Artemidorus's *enhypnion*—dreams arising from bodily states, emotional turbulence, or recent waking experience. These carry no prophetic value and require no interpretation beyond recognizing their somatic or psychological source.

*Visum* or *phantasma* (apparition): The image seen in the hypnagogic state between waking and sleeping. These are not true dreams but threshold phenomena—faces, forms, sounds that appear as consciousness transitions. Later Persian tradition would treat certain *phantasma* experiences as significant (the 'ecstatic visions' of the Turning of the Soul), but Macrobius generally dismissed them as insignificant.

Of these five, only the first three warrant interpretive attention. The *somnium* requires symbolic analysis. The *visio* requires recognition and preparation. The *oraculum* requires response to divine instruction. The last two are noise rather than signal.

## The Soul's Descent

Macrobius located dream experience within the Neoplatonic cosmology of the soul's descent through planetary spheres. Before incarnation, the soul dwells in pure celestial light. As it descends toward earthly embodiment, it passes through each planetary sphere in turn, acquiring specific capacities from each: reason from Saturn, the power to act from Jupiter, bold spirit from Mars, sense-perception and imagination from the Sun, desire from Venus, the capacity to articulate from Mercury, and the power to generate physical form from the Moon.

Dreams reverse this descent. Sleep loosens the body's hold; the soul rises toward what it remembers. During sleep, the soul partially withdraws from bodily engagement and reascends toward its celestial origin. The quality of dreams depends on how far the soul rises. Dreams trapped in the lunar sphere reflect bodily concerns (*insomnium*). Dreams reaching the solar sphere gain clarity and prophetic power. Dreams touching the higher spheres may receive direct divine communication (*oraculum*).

This framework explains why dream quality varies. The soul encumbered by bodily disturbance cannot rise far; its dreams remain somatic. The soul that has purified itself through philosophical practice or ritual preparation ascends higher; its dreams touch prophetic sources. The cosmic architecture provides gradations of dream significance corresponding to gradations of celestial access.

## Asclepian Incubation: The Temple of Dreams

If Artemidorus provided method and Macrobius provided cosmology, the cult of Asclepius provided institutional practice. At healing sanctuaries throughout the Greek and Roman world—most famously at Epidaurus—seekers slept in sacred precincts to receive therapeutic dreams. This was not passive hope but structured ritual, a technology for inducing divine encounter.

### *The Procedure*

The seeker arriving at the Asklepion underwent a defined sequence. Purification came first: ritual bathing, dietary restrictions, abstention from wine and certain foods, sometimes fasting. The body had to be prepared as a vessel for divine communication.

*Sacrifice* followed—offerings to Asclepius and the associated deities. The seeker established a relationship with the god, demonstrating piety and intention. Inscriptions at Epidaurus record the offerings made and the dreams received, creating an archive of divine-human exchange.

*Incubation* occurred in the *abaton* (sacred dormitory)—a space forbidden to ordinary access, entered only for the ritual of sacred sleep. The seeker lay down on a *kline* (couch), sometimes on the skin of a sacrificed animal, and waited for the god. Priests may have assisted the transition through chanting, incense, or other techniques that induced receptive states.

*Theophany*—the appearance of the god—was the goal. Asclepius might appear directly, performing healing in the dream itself, or he might send one of his children: Hygieia (Health) or Panacea (All-Healing). Sometimes he appeared in symbolic form—as a serpent, his sacred animal—and the dreamer woke healed. Sometimes he gave instructions: a remedy to prepare, a behavior to change, a further offering to make. The temple priests helped interpret what the god had communicated.

## *Therapeutic Dreams*

The Epidaurian inscriptions record remarkable healings. A man with a paralyzed hand dreams Asclepius bending back his fingers. He wakes. The hand moves. A woman unable to conceive dreams of the god placing a serpent on her belly; she bears a son within the year. A blind man dreams Asclepius opens his eyes; he sees.

Modern readers may interpret these accounts variously—as faith healing, psychosomatic response, temple propaganda, or genuine divine intervention. What matters for the oneiromantic tradition is the framework: dreams can be sought, not merely received; proper preparation increases the likelihood of significant dreams; divine figures can communicate directly through dream imagery; and dream content can have a therapeutic effect.

The Asclepian model persisted. Egyptian temple incubation at sites like Dendara preceded it; Christian dream incubation at saints' shrines continued it. The practice of sleeping in sacred space to receive divine dreams represents one of the most widespread and enduring technologies for accessing the prophetic dimension of sleep.

## The Celestial Framework

Behind Artemidorus's method, Macrobius's cosmology, and Asclepian practice stood the astrological framework that located dreams within celestial architecture. The Hellenistic astrologers did not merely time dreams—they explained why dreams occur, what influences shape them, and how to assess their validity.

### *The Ninth House: Place of the God*

In the Hellenistic house system, each of the twelve houses received not only topics but a name reflecting its essential quality. The ninth house was called *Theos*—God. This was the place where the Sun 'rejoiced,' according to the doctrine of planetary joys. The Sun, representing clarity, consciousness, and truth, found its proper home in the house of divine revelation, prophecy, and philosophical inquiry.

The ninth house sits in the cadent quadrant of the upper hemisphere, past the culminating tenth. It represents what lies beyond the visible peak—the transcendent, the foreign, the divine. Long journeys belong here because they take us beyond the familiar. Higher learning belongs here because it takes the mind beyond ordinary knowing. Dreams belong here because they take consciousness beyond waking limits into the territory of the gods.

A natal chart with planets in the ninth house, particularly the luminaries, indicates a soul porous to transcendent insight. The Sun in the ninth suggests one who receives clear, oracular dreams—the *visio* and *oraculum* of Macrobius's taxonomy. The Moon in the ninth suggests one who mediates between celestial and terrestrial realms, translating divine light into imaginal form.

## *The Twelfth House: Bad Spirit*

The twelfth house received a grimmer name: *Kakos Daimon*—Bad Spirit. Where the ninth opens upward toward divine light, the twelfth opens downward toward what is hidden, confined, and feared. This is the house of prisons, hospitals, hidden enemies, self-undoing, and of dreams that arise from disturbance rather than revelation.

Dreams associated with the twelfth house are Macrobius's *insomnium*: nightmares, anxiety dreams, somatic disturbances. They reflect the dreamer's fears, illnesses, and unprocessed psychological material. They require not prophetic interpretation but recognition of their source in the dreamer's own shadows.

The distinction between ninth-house and twelfth-house dreams parallels every tradition's recognition that not all dreams carry equal weight. The question facing the interpreter—does this dream prophesy or merely process?—finds its celestial correlate in the house emphasis of the dream chart or the natal chart's predisposition.

## *The Moon: Giver of Form*

If the ninth house provides the cosmic location for prophetic dreams, the Moon provides the mechanism. Hellenistic cosmology understood the Moon as the boundary between the celestial and sublunary realms. Above the Moon, eternal order; below, change and generation. The Moon translates—she receives the abstract light of the higher spheres and shapes it into the forms of earthly experience.

This makes the Moon the natural ruler of dreams. During sleep, consciousness withdraws from sensory engagement and becomes receptive—lunar in quality. The Moon governs this receptive state and determines what impressions it receives. Her condition in the natal chart indicates the quality of the dreamer's dream life: a well-placed Moon suggests clear, coherent, potentially prophetic dreams; an afflicted Moon suggests confused, disturbing, or unreliable dreams.

The Moon's phase matters. A waxing Moon—increasing in light—is more constructive, capable of bringing visions toward manifestation. A waning Moon is more reflective, better suited to dreams of release or completion. The Moon's aspects to other planets color dream content: Moon-Venus produces 'sweet dreams' of beauty and connection; Moon-Saturn produces dreams of restriction, coldness, or ancestral weight; Moon-Mercury produces dreams of messages, travel, and communication. The Moon colors everything she touches. So do dreams.

## The Hermetic Lots

The Hellenistic tradition developed mathematical points called Lots (later 'Arabic Parts') to isolate specific life themes within the chart. These are calculated by measuring the arc between two planets and projecting that distance from the Ascendant. The resulting point concentrates the relationship between those two planets into a single sensitive degree.

### *A lot of Fortune and Lot of Spirit*

The two fundamental Lots are Fortune and Spirit. The Lot of Fortune relates to the body, material circumstances, and what happens to the native—the passive dimension of fate. The Lot of Spirit relates to the soul, intention, and what the native does—the active dimension of will.

For a day chart (Sun above the horizon): Lot of Fortune = Ascendant + Moon − Sun. Lot of Spirit = Ascendant + Sun − Moon.

For a night chart (Sun below the horizon): the formulas reverse.

Dreams arising from the Lot of Fortune reflect bodily states and material circumstances—the *insomnium* of somatic disturbance. Dreams arising from the Lot of Spirit reflect the soul's purpose and divine intention—the *somnium, visio,* and *oraculum* of prophetic communication. Assessing which Lot is activated helps determine which type of dream the interpreter faces.

### *The Lot of Dreams*

A specific Lot of Dreams (*Pars Somniorum*) appears in some Hellenistic and Persian sources. The most consistent formula takes the distance from the lord of the ninth house to Mercury and projects it from the Ascendant. The logic: Mercury is the messenger of the gods, the translator of divine communication into comprehensible form. His relationship to the ninth-house lord (the planet ruling the place of prophecy) indicates how effectively the native receives and processes dream messages.

If the Lot of Dreams falls in an angular house (first, fourth, seventh, or tenth), dreams carry weight and tend toward manifestation. If it falls in a cadent house (third, sixth, ninth, or twelfth), dreams may be vivid but less likely to produce concrete results. The condition of the Lot's ruler further refines the assessment.

## Chronocrators: When Dreams Activate

The natal chart describes potential; timing techniques determine when that potential activates. Hellenistic and Persian astrologers developed elaborate systems of 'chronocrators' (time-lords) to divide life into periods ruled by specific planets.

### *Annual Profections*

Profections rotate the chart one sign per year. At birth, the Ascendant is emphasized. At age one, the second house. At age two, the third. The cycle repeats every twelve years.

Ninth-house profection years—ages 8, 20, 32, 44, 56, 68—activate the prophetic house. During these years, the native experiences heightened dream activity, clearer prophetic content, and greater access to the *theos* dimension. The planet ruling the ninth house becomes 'Lord of the Year,' and its natal condition and current transits shape the year's dream quality.

Twelfth-house profection years—ages 11, 23, 35, 47, 59, 71—activate the house of hidden disturbance. Dreams during these years may be more troubled, reflecting the native's shadow material, hidden fears, or psychological processing. A malefic ruling the twelfth intensifies this tendency.

### *Firdaria*

The Persian *firdaria* system assigns fixed planetary periods across the lifespan. For a day birth: Sun (10 years), Venus (8 years), Mercury (13 years), Moon (9 years), Saturn (11 years), Jupiter (12 years), Mars (7 years). For a night birth, the sequence begins with Moon.

A native in a Moon *firdar* experiences heightened receptivity, emotional intensity, and vivid dreams. A native in a Mercury *firdar* experiences increased message-dreams, symbolic communication, and mental activity during sleep. The *firdar* lord sets the 'chapter theme' within which dream experiences unfold.

### *The Turning of the Soul*

A specialized Persian technique identifies seven-year cycles when the 'Lord of the Turn' (based on the planetary hour of birth) aligns with the ruler of the Moon's natal mansion. These moments are called 'Turnings of the Soul'—peak windows for active or ecstatic visions, dreams of transformation, and encounters with guiding figures.

The seven-year interval echoes across traditions: the Vedic recognition of major life transitions at multiples of seven, the Western sense of developmental stages, and the body's cellular renewal. At these thresholds, the soul is particularly accessible to dream communication.

## The Arabic Preservation

The Hellenistic synthesis might have been lost had Arabic scholars not preserved and extended it during the centuries when Europe forgot its classical inheritance. Abū Ma'shar (787–886) and other Arabic astrologers translated Greek and Persian texts, developed new techniques, and integrated astrological dream interpretation with the Islamic prophetic tradition.

The ḥadīth literature treats a believer's true dream as one forty-sixth part of prophecy—not full revelation, but a genuine channel to the unseen. Ibn Sīrīn of Basra (653–729) compiled the most influential Islamic dream dictionary, emphasizing that the dreamer's spiritual state affects the dream's significance. A pious person's dream carries a different weight than the same dream experienced by one living carelessly.

Ibn Sīrīn also taught that interpretation participates in manifestation. The classic example: a king dreams that all his teeth fall out. One interpreter says, 'All your family will die before you'—and is beaten for delivering bad news. Another interpreter, shown the same dream, says, 'You will outlive all your relatives—blessed with long life.' Same content, different frame. The dream does not arrive with fixed meaning; the interpreter's framing shapes how it manifests.

This teaching carries weight. The interpreter's word bends the dream's unfolding. The dream-interpreter wields real power and bears real responsibility. Meaning is co-created between dream, dreamer, and interpreter.

Through Latin translations of Arabic texts, this integrated tradition—Greek method, Persian timing, Islamic spiritual sensitivity—entered medieval Europe. Guido Bonatti's thirteenth-century *Liber Astronomiae* transmits the Arabic synthesis, providing the protocols that the following chapter examines in detail.

## What the Greeks Synthesized

The Hellenistic achievement was integration. Babylonian omens, Egyptian temple practice, Greek philosophy, and Persian theology merged into a coherent framework where dreams found their place within cosmic order.

**Classification first.** Before interpreting content, determine the dream's type. Is this *oneiros* or *enhypnion*? *Somnium*, *visio*, or *oraculum*? Ninth-house clarity or twelfth-house processing? The same dream requires a different response depending on its category.

**Context always.** Artemidorus insisted: know the dreamer. Occupation, health, status, age, and circumstances—all modify meaning. The dream interpreter who applies fixed symbol-meanings without contextual assessment follows letter rather than spirit.

**Celestial location.** Dreams occur within cosmic architecture. The ninth house and its lord, the Moon and her condition, the activated Lots and chronocrators—these provide the 'where' and 'when' that frame the 'what' of dream content.

**Interpretation participates.** The dream does not arrive complete; meaning emerges through the interpretive encounter. How the interpreter frames the dream affects how it manifests. This power demands responsibility.

**Dreams can be sought.** The Asclepian model demonstrates that significant dreams are not merely random gifts but can be cultivated through preparation, purification, and ritual attention. The practitioner who understands incubation can guide patients toward dreams that provide needed information. The Greeks gave us the questions. Bonatti gave us the method.

## Toward Medieval Practice

The Greek synthesis provided the framework. The Arabic preservation ensured its survival. What remained was practical application—a working method for the dream-interpreter who sits with a client's dream and must assess its significance, identify its celestial correlates, and offer guidance that serves the dreamer's flourishing.

Guido Bonatti, writing in thirteenth-century Italy, provided exactly this. His *Liber Astronomiae* devotes an entire treatise to dreams: how to cast the dream chart, identify the significator, read the houses for subject matter, and apply essential dignities to assess whether the dream speaks true. Where the Greeks provided theory, Bonatti provided protocol.

The chapter that follows examines Bonatti's method in detail—the ninth-house emphasis, the validation criteria, the house-by-house analysis of dream content. The Hellenistic inheritance meets medieval practice. The reunion of streams continues its flow toward the present day.

# Sources

Artemidorus of Daldis. *Oneirocritica*. Translated by Robert J. White. Park Ridge: Noyes Press, 1975.

Edelstein, Emma J., and Ludwig Edelstein. *Asclepius: Collection and Interpretation of the Testimonies*. 2 vols. Baltimore: Johns Hopkins University Press, 1945.

Macrobius. *Commentary on the Dream of Scipio*. Translated by William Harris Stahl. New York: Columbia University Press, 1952.

Meier, C. A. *Healing Dream and Ritual: Ancient Incubation and Modern Psychotherapy*. Einsiedeln: Daimon Verlag, 1989.

Dorotheus of Sidon. *Carmen Astrologicum*. Translated by Benjamin N. Dykes. Minneapolis: Cazimi Press, 2017.

Valens, Vettius. *Anthologies*. Translated by Mark Riley. 2010. Available at csus.edu/indiv/r/rileymt/.

Firmicus Maternus. *Mathesis*. Translated by Jean Rhys Bram as *Ancient Astrology Theory and Practice*. Park Ridge: Noyes Press, 1975.

Ibn Sīrīn. *Tafsīr al-Aḥlām al-Kabīr*. Various editions and translations.

Bonatti, Guido. *Liber Astronomiae*. Translated by Benjamin N. Dykes. Minneapolis: Cazimi Press, 2007.

## Chapter Eleven

# Persian and Arabic Dream Astrology

*al-ru'yā al-ṣāliḥa juz'un min sittatin wa-arba'īna juz'an min al-nubuwwa*

*The true dream is one forty-sixth part of prophecy.*

—Ḥadīth, Ṣaḥīḥ al-Bukhārī

On the external-internal spectrum, the Persian-Arabic synthesis stands midway—but with distinctive emphasis on the dreamer's moral condition. The dream remains external communication—prophetic message descending through celestial hierarchy from the Active Intellect—but reception depends on the soul's alignment with divine order. Ibn Sīrīn's insight that the same symbol signifies differently for different spiritual states parallels Egyptian constitutional typology while adding an ethical dimension. The tradition preserves external sourcing while recognizing that internal purification determines reception quality.

## Beyond Transmission

The Persians and Arabs did not preserve the Greek inheritance. They transformed it. While Europe forgot, scholars under Sassanid and Islamic patronage translated, refined, and reframed the Hellenistic synthesis. Not reproduction—development. New timing techniques. New theological frameworks. New understanding of how celestial influence reaches the sleeping mind.

Greece provided method (Artemidorus), cosmology (Macrobius), and institutional practice (the Asklepieia). Persia added emanationist theology—the Active Intellect as source of celestial communication—and chronocratoria dividing life into planetary chapters. Islam added prophetic validation—the dream as fractional prophecy—and an ethics recognizing the interpreter's power to shape manifestation.

What Guido Bonatti received in thirteenth-century Italy was not raw Hellenistic astrology. It was Greek mathematics clothed in Persian cosmology and refined by Arabic scholarship. To understand medieval European dream astrology, start here.

## The Sassanid Context

The Sassanid Empire (224–651 CE) gathered what had scattered. Shāpūr I and Khosrow I viewed gathering scientific knowledge from Greece, India, and Mesopotamia as a religious duty. They believed these traditions were fragments of original Zoroastrian wisdom scattered by Alexander's conquests. Translation into Pahlavi was not passive preservation but active reshaping to align with Iranian theology.

Dorotheus of Sidon, Vettius Valens, and Ptolemy—they entered Persian intellectual culture transformed. Hellenistic precision and fate merged with Zoroastrian dualism: the cosmic battle between Ahura Mazda (the Wise Lord) and Angra Mainyu (the Destructive Spirit).

## *The Theological Reframing*

The celestial firmament was a battlefield. Zodiacal constellations and luminaries—soldiers of Ahura Mazda maintaining cosmic order (*Asha*). The planets—wandering stars moving irregularly against the fixed background—demonic entities (*pairikās*) that had broken through celestial ramparts to sow discord.

This gave oneiromancy moral urgency. A dream was not merely a message but a potential site of spiritual warfare. Divine revelation—or demonic deception. Which influence prevailed depended on the celestial forces dominant at the time of sleep. Assessment required knowing not just what was dreamed but under whose stars.

## *The Architecture of Ascent*

Zoroastrian cosmology provided the vertical hierarchy. The heavens are divided into stations: stars, Moon, Sun, and finally the Endless Lights (Anaghran), closest to Ahura Mazda's abode. Later Pahlavi sources elaborated sevenfold models influenced by Greek planetary theory.

The spiritual realm (*mēnōg*) connects to the material realm (*gētīg*) through celestial emanations. Dreams occur when the soul temporarily returns to *mēnōg* during sleep. Access to *bāṭen* (inner knowledge) requires purification—the soul must reflect higher emanations without interference from demonic wandering stars.

This anticipates Macrobius's Neoplatonic ladder and the Arabic Active Intellect doctrine. The Persian contribution: embedding celestial ascent within a moral cosmology where dream quality depends on the soul's alignment with divine order.

## Persian Innovations: The Chapters of Life

The Persians developed chronocratoria—time-lord systems—beyond anything the Greeks achieved. Life divided into planetary chapters. Each ruled by a specific celestial body whose natal condition determines the chapter's quality.

### *The Firdaria*

The firdaria (from Persian *al-firdariya,* derived from Greek *periodos*) operates on a fixed 75-year cycle. Nine major periods ruled by the seven classical planets and the two lunar nodes. Sequence depends on sect—day birth (Sun leads) or night birth (Moon leads).

*Table 11.1. Firdaria Periods by Sect*

| Planet/Node | Years | Diurnal Order | Nocturnal Order |
|---|---|---|---|
| Sun | 10 | 1st (ages 0–10) | 5th (ages 39–49) |
| Venus | 8 | 2nd (ages 10–18) | 6th (ages 49–57) |
| Mercury | 13 | 3rd (ages 18–31) | 7th (ages 57–70) |
| Moon | 9 | 4th (ages 31–40) | 1st (ages 0–9) |
| Saturn | 11 | 5th (ages 40–51) | 2nd (ages 9–20) |
| Jupiter | 12 | 6th (ages 51–63) | 3rd (ages 20–32) |
| Mars | 7 | 7th (ages 63–70) | 4th (ages 32–39) |
| North Node | 3 | 8th (ages 70–73) | 8th (ages 70–73) |
| South Node | 2 | 9th (ages 73–75) | 9th (ages 73–75) |

Each major period subdivides into seven sub-periods following Chaldean order. The ruling planet's natal condition—dignity, house placement, aspects—determines whether the chapter brings benefit or difficulty.

For dream interpretation, the firdaria is macro-filter. A dream of royal power during Sun firdar suggests literal success. Same dream during Saturn firdar—heavy responsibility, approaching decline. Moon firdar heightens dream receptivity and emotional intensity. Dreams during Moon periods carry particular weight.

### *The Turning of the Soul*

Complementing firdaria: the Turning of the Soul, based on the Lord of the Turn (*sāl-khudā*). A planetary ruler assigned to each year of life based on the planetary hour of birth. First year ruled by birth-hour planet; subsequent years follow Chaldean order perpetually.

Great Turn: every seven years as the cycle completes rotation through the seven planets. The specific Turning of the Soul occurs when Lord of the Turn coincides with lord of Moon's natal mansion. Peak windows for psychic transformation—times when the soul realigns with celestial origin.

Dreams during a Turning were treated with exceptional gravity. Active visions, ecstatic experiences at these thresholds—dreams of miraculous powers, guiding figures, departure from the body. The seven-year interval echoes everywhere: Vedic stages, Western cellular renewal, the sense that life moves through chapters. At these thresholds, the soul is accessible.

## Dreams and Royal Legitimation

*Farra-ye Kayānī*—the Divine Glory, Royal Splendor. A luminous force validating the right to rule. Astral signature of legitimacy. Described as radiant light or symbolic creature—ram, great bird—accompanying the chosen ruler.

Dreams were the primary medium through which *farr* was manifested or confirmed. A king receiving true vision possessed divine glory. Loss of *farr* was typically preceded by fragmented or demonic dreams. Court Oneirocriticism emerged—the chief astrologer (*mowbed*) analyzed royal dreams to assess stability of state.

The Nine Dreams of the King of Qannūj illustrates this practice. Bizarre images—white elephant chased by black dog, river made of fire—decoded as specific political threats and opportunities. Not private spiritual counsel but public declaration of the state's celestial alignment.

The king's access to *bāṭen* was requirement of office. By correctly interpreting celestial messages, the king demonstrated alignment with the Active Intellect, ensuring justice (*Dād*) in the material realm. Dream interpretation became statecraft. The king who read dreams correctly ruled correctly.

# The Islamic Prophetic Framework

The transition from Sassanid to Islamic rule integrated Persian astrological doctrines into monotheistic framework. Cornerstone of Islamic oneiromancy: the ḥadīth stating that a good dream (*ru'ya ṣādiqa*) is one part of forty-six parts of prophecy.

## *The Rationale of the Fraction*

Historical-mathematical rationale for this specific ratio: Muhammad received divine inspiration through true dreams six months before the first Quranic revelation at the Cave of Hira. His prophetic mission lasted twenty-three years. Six months is one forty-sixth of twenty-three years. The true dream—initial, preparatory stage of revelation.

This elevated the true dream to certainty. A message from the unseen (*ghayb*) requiring the same interpretive care as scripture. Not psychological phenomenon but fractional prophecy—genuine access to divine knowledge through a channel that remained open after the seal of prophecy.

## *The Three Types of Dreams*

Islamic tradition categorized dreams into three types based on origin.

*Ru'ya* (the true dream): Also *ru'ya ṣādiqa* or *bushrā* (glad tidings). Originates from God or angels. Clarity, internal coherence, fulfillment—comes true like bright daylight. Occurs near dawn. Leaves lasting impression. Concerns matters beyond ordinary knowledge.

*Ḥulm* (the satanic dream): Distressing visions sent by Shayṭān to terrify or misguide. Fear, confusion, jumbled narratives. Response: spit three times to the left, seek refuge in Allah, do not discuss with others. Requires protection, not interpretation.

*Ḥadīth al-nafs* (talk of the self): Psychological dreams reflecting waking thoughts, desires, worries, bodily states. Dreaming of water when thirsty. Dreaming of exam when anxious. Requires neither prophetic interpretation nor protective response—only recognition of mundane source.

This parallels Macrobius (*oraculum/insomnium/visum*) and the Vedic *bhāvika/doṣaja* distinction. Traditions converge: not all dreams are equal. Classification precedes interpretation.

# Ibn Sīrīn: The Ethics of Interpretation

Muhammad Ibn Sīrīn (653–728 CE) compiled the most influential Islamic dream dictionary, the *Tafsīr al-Aḥlām al-Kabīr*. But his method moved far beyond dictionary lookup. Dynamic, context-dependent analysis placing the dreamer's spiritual state at center.

## *The Dreamer as Primary Filter*

Ibn Sīrīn's critical insight: a dream symbol has no fixed meaning. Interpretation depends entirely on spiritual state (*ḥāl*) of the dreamer. Rope might signify covenant with God for the pious—bondage or debt for the worldly. Same image, different souls, different significance.

This parallels Artemidorus on knowing the dreamer's occupation and circumstances—but adds spiritual dimension. Not just social position but moral condition shapes meaning. Ibn Sīrīn warned: dream interpretation is religious act. Look well from whom you take your religion!

Clinical implication: the interpreter must assess not only celestial timing and symbolic content but the dreamer's character, circumstances, spiritual orientation. A dream of illumination for someone actively pursuing wisdom differs fundamentally from the same dream in spiritual crisis.

### *Interpretation Participates in Manifestation*

Ibn Sīrīn taught that interpretation participates in fulfillment. The ḥadīth: a dream is on the wing of a bird until interpreted—suspended, awaiting the word that grounds it into reality. How the interpreter frames the vision determines how it unfolds.

Classical example: a king dreams all his teeth fall out. One interpreter says, All your family will die before you. The king has him beaten. Another interpreter, same dream: You will outlive all your relatives—blessed with long life. Same content. Different frame. Both true—emphasizing different aspects of the same symbolic complex. But the first grounds loss; the second grounds longevity.

This teaching carries weight. The dream does not arrive with fixed meaning. Meaning emerges through the interpretive encounter. The interpreter wields real power, bears real responsibility. Framing must serve the dreamer's flourishing while remaining honest about content.

Ibn Sīrīn was known for extreme caution. He often refused to interpret distressing dreams, preferring silence to grounding negative outcomes. Not evasion—ethical practice. The interpreter is participant, not observer.

## Abū Ma'shar and the Astrological Synthesis

Ja'far ibn Muḥammad Abū Ma'shar al-Balkhī (787–886 CE) brought Persian and Arabic streams into systematic integration. Coming from Balkh (center of Persian culture) to Baghdad, he became primary architect of the astrological frameworks that would reach medieval Europe.

## *The Active Intellect*

Abū Ma'shar and philosophers like al-Fārābī and Ibn Sīnā used Neoplatonic emanationism to explain how celestial images reach the mind. The universe emanates from the First Cause through ten successive intellects. The tenth—the Active Intellect (*al-'aql al-fa''āl*)—rules the sublunary sphere as giver of forms.

The human imagination (*mutakhayyila*) stores sensory forms and recombines them endlessly. During sleep, senses dormant, imagination receives intelligible truths from the Active Intellect. But the soul is habituated to the physical world—imagination clothes abstract truths in sensible forms. Symbols resembling material objects but carrying higher reality.

This explains both why dreams are symbolic (imagination translates abstract truth into concrete imagery) and why interpretation is necessary (the symbol must be traced to its intelligible source). The dream is structured communication, limited only by imagination's capacity to receive and translate.

## *Planetary Metaphors*

Abū Ma'shar's *Astrological Metaphors* provided bridges between chart mathematics and dream imagery. Anthropomorphic and social analogies explaining planetary combinations—shorthand the dream interpreter could apply directly.

Venus with Mars: a woman seeking pleasure who joins a perverse man; she fears him but pretends affection. In dreams: coerced agreement, hidden anxiety in relationship. Venus with Saturn: young woman with good figure keeping company with old, impotent man; distressed, life unbearable. Jupiter with Mars: honest man joining wicked and dissolute one.

These metaphors translate planetary configurations into narrative scenes—scripts the dreamer's subconscious might follow. Dream chart shows Venus-Mars contact, dream involves attraction mixed with fear: the planetary metaphor illuminates both source and significance.

## The Moon Doctrine

Arabic astrologers made the Moon primary significator of dreams. Closest to the sublunary realm. Collector of light from all other planets. Mediator between celestial influence and earthly manifestation. Her condition in dream chart—or natal chart—determines dream quality fundamentally.

The tradition identified seventeen impediments weakening the Moon, potentially invalidating a dream or inquiry.

*Table 11.2. Selected Lunar Impediments*

| Impediment | Description | Dream Implication |
|---|---|---|
| Combust | Within 15° of Sun (applying) or 12° (separating) | Message hidden or burnt out |
| Void of Course | Making no aspect before leaving sign | Dream is feral; no event follows |
| *Via Combusta* | Between 15° Libra and 15° Scorpio | Extreme instability; caution |
| Besieged | Between Mars and Saturn | Soul under attack; likely *ḥulm* |
| In Fall | Moon in Scorpio | Diminished receptivity |
| Slow in Course | Moving less than average daily motion | Delayed manifestation |

Moon suffering multiple impediments: the dream lacks prophetic weight. Belongs to *ḥulm* or *ḥadīth al-nafs* categories rather than *ru'ya*. Well-dignified Moon in good aspect to benefics: dream channel is clear, message reliable.

# Transmission to Europe

The doctrines of Abū Ma'shar, Māshā'allāh, and Ibn Sīrīn reached medieval Europe through twelfth- and thirteenth-century translation movements centered in Toledo and Sicily. Arabic texts became Latin texts. Persian frameworks became European practice.

Guido Bonatti's *Liber Astronomiae* (c. 1277) is the primary repository. Bonatti preserved the Arabic Moon doctrine—including the seventeen impediments—as foundation for horary and natal interpretation. He maintained Arabic terminology: *Alchecohol* for profection, *Alatifall* for conjunction. Most significantly: the ninth-house doctrine as locus of dreams and higher knowledge.

What Bonatti received was not raw Hellenistic astrology but the transformed tradition. Greek precision refined by Persian theology and Arabic scholarship. The emphasis on the dreamer's interior state, the recognition that interpretation participates in manifestation, the sophisticated timing techniques—all entered European practice through this transmission.

## What the Persian and Arabic Traditions Teach

Life has chapters. The firdaria divides life into planetary chapters. Dreams during a particular firdar carry that planet's signature. A Saturn-period dream addresses different concerns than a Venus-period dream, even if the imagery superficially resembles.

Seven-year thresholds matter. The Turning of the Soul identifies peak windows for transformative dreams. Track seven-year intervals from birth—and from other significant beginnings—as times when the dream channel opens wider.

The dreamer's state filters meaning. Ibn Sīrīn's insight: spiritual condition shapes interpretation. The same dream content requires a different response depending on who dreams it. Assessment must include character and circumstances, not only celestial timing.

Interpretation participates. The dream suspended on the wing of a bird awaits the word that grounds it. Frame the teeth-falling dream as loss—loss manifests. Frame it as longevity—longevity manifests. Both true readings. The choice is ethical as well as technical.

Classification precedes interpretation. The threefold typology—*ru'ya, ḥulm, ḥadīth al-nafs*—parallels every tradition's recognition: not all dreams warrant the same response. Prophetic analysis applied to anxiety processing wastes effort. Divine communication dismissed as psychology misses the message.

The Moon governs reception. Her condition determines whether the dream channel is clear or obstructed. The seventeen impediments provide specific criteria. Afflicted Moon—less weight. Well-dignified Moon in good aspect to benefics—reliable. The channel is open. Listen.

## Toward Medieval Practice

The Persian and Arabic traditions provided theoretical framework. What remained: practical protocol. The step-by-step method for the dream interpreter facing an actual dream.

Guido Bonatti supplied exactly this. His treatment of dreams in the *Liber Astronomiae* provides working method: how to cast the dream chart, identify the significator, read houses for subject matter, apply essential dignities to assess veracity. Where Persians and Arabs provided theology and timing, Bonatti provided procedure.

The chapter that follows examines Bonatti's ninth-house protocols in detail. The reunion of streams continues—from Babylon through Alexandria, through Ctesiphon and Baghdad, through Toledo, finally reaching the Italian astrologer whose practical manual shaped European dream interpretation for centuries.

## Sources

Abū Ma'shar. *The Abbreviation of the Introduction to Astrology*. Translated by Charles Burnett. Leiden: Brill, 1994.

Abū Ma'shar. *On Historical Astrology: The Book of Religions and Dynasties*. Translated by Keiji Yamamoto and Charles Burnett. Leiden: Brill, 2000.

Al-Bīrūnī. *The Book of Instruction in the Elements of the Art of Astrology*. Translated by R. Ramsay Wright. London: Luzac, 1934.

Bonatti, Guido. *Liber Astronomiae*. Translated by Benjamin N. Dykes. Minneapolis: Cazimi Press, 2007.

Dorotheus of Sidon. *Carmen Astrologicum*. Translated by Benjamin N. Dykes. Minneapolis: Cazimi Press, 2017.

Ibn Sīrīn. *Tafsīr al-Aḥlām al-Kabīr*. Various editions.

Pingree, David. *From Astral Omens to Astrology: From Babylon to Bīkāner*. Rome: Istituto Italiano per l'Africa e l'Oriente, 1997.

Stoyanov, Yuri. *The Other God: Dualist Religions from Antiquity to the Cathar Heresy*. New Haven: Yale University Press, 2000.

Zaehner, R. C. *The Dawn and Twilight of Zoroastrianism*. London: Weidenfeld and Nicolson, 1961.

## Part Three

# Integration and Practice

*Visita Interiora Terrae Rectificando Invenies Occultum Lapidem*

**"Visit the interior of the earth; by rectifying you will find the hidden stone."**

—Alchemical axiom (V.I.T.R.I.O.L.)

Synthesis is not collection. The traditions surveyed in Part Two do not automatically combine; their integration requires work—the opus that transforms inherited knowledge into living practice.

The three chapters that follow accomplish this integration. Chapter Twelve recovers the Latin reception of Arabic dream astrology, centering on Guido Bonatti's ninth-house protocols for assessing dream veracity. Chapter Thirteen weaves the cultural transmissions into a unified clinical methodology—the threefold assessment combining Western astrological, Vedic, and Chinese medical frameworks. Chapter Fourteen completes the arc with the materia medica of dream work: the plant allies that open gates, clarify vision, and preserve what the dreamer brings back.

Work against nature—not opposition but completion. The dream arrives unbidden. What we do with it is craft.

## Chapter Twelve

# The Latin Reception

## *The Ninth House and Dream Veracity*

*θεῖον γάρ τι καὶ τὸ ἐνύπνιον*

*For the dream is something divine.*

—Aristotle, On Divination in Sleep 463b

Bonatti's protocols ask a different question. Not where the dream comes from—external message or internal processing—but whether this dream is true. Veracity assessment cuts across the spectrum. Divine communication, organ-spirit activity, anything between: essential dignities and lunar testimony assess reliability regardless of source. This chapter provides the filter that Western astrological practice uses to distinguish signal from noise.

## The Domus Dei

The ninth house carries associations with prophecy, divine communication, and higher knowledge since the Hellenistic period. Vettius Valens: travel, foreign lands, prophecy, divine matters. Medieval astrologers called it the *Domus Dei*—House of God. Where human consciousness touches what lies beyond.

Ptolemy assigned the ninth to long journeys and religion. Firmicus Maternus expanded: dreams, visions, divination—seers, diviners, prophets, dream interpreters. The logic coheres. All ninth house matters extend beyond ordinary perception. Long journeys carry us past familiar territory. Religion addresses realities beyond material demonstration. Dreams transport us beyond waking consciousness.

Previous chapters traced oneiromancy through cultural streams—Mesopotamian, Egyptian, Vedic, Chinese, Bön, Greek, Persian, Arabic. Each developed within its own cosmological structure. Each asks different questions of a dream. This chapter provides the Western astrological apparatus: where prophetic dreams enter (the ninth house) and how to assess reliability (Bonatti's veracity protocols).

### *Cadent House Dynamics*

The ninth occupies a cadent position, declining from the angular tenth at the Midheaven. The cadent houses—third, sixth, ninth, twelfth—take their name from Latin *cadens*: falling. Traditional astrology considered them weaker than angular or succedent placements for manifesting concrete results. Apparent weakness conceals different strength.

Cadent houses govern mental operations preceding action. The ninth receives inspiration; the tenth manifests it publicly. Hellenistic astrologers named this place *Theos*—the God. Insight gestates here before taking visible form.

The ninth stands in trine to the Ascendant—120 degrees. Ptolemy calls the trine harmonious because it connects signs of the same gender. Squares generate tension; oppositions polarize. The trine opens unobstructed channel. Dreamer and dream flow together. Prophetic content integrates readily into waking awareness.

### *Joy of the Sun*

The ninth serves as joy of the Sun—the position where that luminary finds natural home and expresses significations most freely. Bonatti in the *Liber Astronomiae*: the ninth house, as joy of the Sun, illuminates hidden matters through dreams and divination.

The Sun makes visible what was hidden. Dreams, though experienced in darkness, nonetheless illuminate. They reveal hidden patterns, disclose truths waking consciousness obscures, bring light to shadowed regions of psyche and circumstance. The Sun's joy in the ninth affirms this revelatory function.

## Triplicity Lords and the Lord of Divination

Each zodiacal sign belongs to one of four elemental triplicities. Three planetary lords govern each, assigned according to sect. Dorotheus of Sidon establishes this system in the *Carmen Astrologicum*.

*Table 12.1. Triplicity Lords by Element*

| Triplicity | Signs | Day Lord | Night Lord | Participating |
|---|---|---|---|---|
| Fire | Aries, Leo, Sagittarius | Sun | Jupiter | Saturn |
| Earth | Taurus, Virgo, Capricorn | Venus | Moon | Mars |
| Air | Gemini, Libra, Aquarius | Saturn | Mercury | Jupiter |
| Water | Cancer, Scorpio, Pisces | Venus | Mars | Moon |

Traditional practice assigns the three triplicity lords to successive life periods. First lord—determined by sect, diurnal for day charts, nocturnal for night—governs roughly the first third of life. Second lord governs middle years. Third—the participating lord—governs final phase and reveals outcome.

Applied to the ninth house, these three lords trace the arc of prophetic capacity across the lifespan. Strong first lord: early receptivity to significant dreams. Strong second lord: divinatory faculty develops during mature years. Third lord—bearing the title Lord of Divination—reveals whether prophetic gifts ultimately flower or wither.

The planet shapes the gift. Saturn as Lord of Divination brings dreams of duration: ancestral patterns, karmic weight, what unfolds across years. Jupiter opens channels of guidance and teaching. Mars cuts to conflict and action. Essential dignity governs clarity. In domicile or exaltation, meaning arrives accessible; the channel runs clear. Peregrine, messages scatter with nothing to ground them. Afflicted by malefic without reception, dreams come heavy and hard to absorb.

## Elemental Signatures

The element of the sign on the ninth house cusp colors dream quality and the mode through which prophetic information enters.

*Table 12.2. Elemental Dream Qualities*

| Element | Dream Quality | Manifestation | Challenge |
|---|---|---|---|
| Fire | Heroic, bright | Direct commands | Courage to act |
| Earth | Grounded, material | Practical warnings | Verification of facts |
| Air | Symbolic, verbal | Puzzles, language | Over-analysis |
| Water | Emotional, numinous | Feelings, spirits | Distinguishing projection |

Fire signs on the ninth (Aries, Leo, Sagittarius): dreams of quest, battle, spiritual illumination. The dreamer experiences command or revelation. The challenge lies not in deciphering obscure symbolism but in mustering courage to follow direction given.

Earth signs (Taurus, Virgo, Capricorn) ground dreams in practical concern—property, health, work, finances. These dreams seem mundane, but concreteness makes them easier to verify. A dream about finding money in a specific location can be tested; a dream about spiritual enlightenment cannot.

Air signs (Gemini, Libra, Aquarius) generate dreams that communicate through language, symbol, intellectual pattern. Characters speak. Messages appear written. The dreamer wakes with a puzzle to solve rather than an instruction to follow.

Water signs (Cancer, Scorpio, Pisces) open dreams to emotional depths, ancestral memory, psychic attunement. Deceased relatives visit. Numinous encounters resist verbal description. Water sign dreamers may experience genuinely precognitive dreams, telepathic contact, communion with the dead. Challenge: distinguishing psychic content from emotional projection.

## The Tripartite Night

The triplicity principle applies not only to zodiacal signs but to time. The night divides into three watches, each governed by one triplicity lord of the ninth house sign. This synthesizes Hellenistic planetary rulership with timing principles established in Vedic tradition. Varāhamihira's *Bṛhat Saṃhitā* establishes the foundational doctrine; see Chapter Five for full Jyotiṣa treatment.

*Table 12.3. Dream Timing and Manifestation Period*

| Watch | Approximate Time | Manifestation |
|---|---|---|
| First | Sunset – Midnight | Months to years |
| Second | Midnight – 4:00 AM | Weeks to months |
| Third | 4:00 AM – Sunrise | Days to hours |

Clinical observation adds another layer. First watch processes the day just ended—unfinished business, residual emotion, psyche clearing its desk. Third watch prepares for the day ahead, reflecting anticipatory concerns. Middle watch, freed from backward glance and forward anxiety, opens most reliably to prophetic content. This accords with Varāhamihira: first and third watches carry more noise; oracular signal strengthens around midnight.

The watch shapes message as surely as messenger. Triplicity lords of the ninth house cusp color dreams in each period. Cancer on ninth cusp: first watch falls under Venus (day lord) or Mars (night lord), second under the alternate, third under Moon. First-watch dream carries that lord's coloring; third-watch dream carries lunar themes—nurturing, memory, emotional fluctuation.

### *Practical Application*

Note not only dream content but timing. Train yourself to check the time upon waking from significant dreams—or develop sufficient awareness to note approximate time within the dream itself. Urgency, manifestation timeline, thematic coloring: all depend partly on when during the night the dream occurred.

Know your natal ninth house. Develop a personalized map of nocturnal territory. Which triplicity lord governs each watch? Dreams consistently occurring during Saturn's watch address different themes than those during Jupiter's watch, even when surface content seems similar. Timing reveals planetary signature underlying the message.

## Horary Applications

Natal astrology reveals general prophetic capacity. Horary interprets specific dreams. Cast a chart for moment of waking, moment of recollection, or moment of recounting in consultation. Each captures valid celestial configuration. Ninth house becomes primary focus.

Ascendant represents the dreamer. Ninth house cusp and its lord represent the dream. Strong reception between first and ninth house rulers: dream arrives as a gift, readily grasped. Mutual aversion—signs sharing no Ptolemaic aspect—blocks access. The message comes; the dreamer cannot reach it.

Planets in the ninth color dream content. Mars: conflict. Venus: pleasure and relationship. Ninth house ruler's essential dignity reveals fundamental quality—domicile brings clarity; peregrine scatters. House placement shows where message applies; aspects reveal what forces shape it.

Moon serves as general significator—association with night, unconscious, receptive states. Moon applying to Jupiter: opportunity. Applying to Saturn: limitations, responsibilities. Moon making no close aspects: dream stands alone, unconnected to developing circumstances.

Mercury takes co-rulership when dreams contain speech, writing, numbers, symbolic puzzles—the messenger god translates between registers, rendering celestial pattern into human language. Mercury well-placed: dreamer wakes with words for what they saw. Mercury afflicted or combust: message arrives but language fails it. Dream slips back into silence.

## Dreams and Contemplative Visions

These tools apply equally to visions arising in meditation, prayer, contemplative absorption. Contemplative practice produces the same phenomena: voices, visions, presence events. Single channel, various entry points.

Abraham Abulafia induced visions through letter permutation and breath. Isaac of Akko received revelations at the hypnagogic threshold—same liminal space dreams occupy. Al-Ghazālī treated dreams and intuitive insights as single category. Buddhist *jhānas* parallel lucid dream awareness. Teresa of Ávila's sixth-mansion visions arrive through stillness, not sleep, yet require the same discernment. Abhinavagupta's 112 *dhāraṇās* open portals indistinguishable from dream gates.

The ninth house governs dreams and visions alike. Lord of Divination indicates prophetic capacity whether native sleeps or sits. Sleep relaxes the threshold; contemplative practice crosses it deliberately. Celestial assessment holds either way.

# The Problem of Veracity

Every dream interpreter faces the same challenge: distinguishing significant from insignificant dreams. Divine communication demands serious attention; indigestion deserves only a change in diet. Guido Bonatti developed systematic protocols for this discrimination. His *Liber Astronomiae*—the most comprehensive medieval Latin treatment of judicial astrology—establishes objective criteria for judging dream veracity.

Bonatti's rules do not replace intuition. They focus it. Before decoding symbols, the dream must pass specific tests. If it fails, the dream may be psychologically interesting. It is not prophecy.

The Persian-Arabic tradition (Chapter Eleven) contributed threefold classification and the ethical principle that interpretation participates in manifestation. Bonatti provides technical criteria: essential dignity, combustion, malefic affliction, reception, lunar testimony. Together, these tools transform dream assessment from impression to method.

# Essential Dignity

Bonatti's system relies on essential dignity—planetary strength by zodiacal position. From Latin *essentia*: what the planet is, not where it happens to be. Five levels: domicile (sign planet rules), exaltation (powers elevated), triplicity (elemental affinity), term (degree segment), face (decanate). Point values: five for domicile, four for exaltation, three for triplicity, two for term, one for face.

## *Domicile and Exaltation*

A planet in its own sign operates with full authority. Sun rules Leo. Moon rules Cancer. Mercury rules Gemini and Virgo. Venus rules Taurus and Libra. Mars rules Aries and Scorpio. Jupiter rules Sagittarius and Pisces. Saturn rules Capricorn and Aquarius. In home positions, each planet signifies with clarity and reliability. Ninth house ruler in domicile: dreams possess inherent truthfulness. The planetary messenger delivers without distortion.

Exaltation confers elevation rather than ownership. Sun exalted in Aries. Moon in Taurus. Mercury in Virgo. Venus in Pisces. Mars in Capricorn. Jupiter in Cancer. Saturn in Libra. Ninth house ruler in exaltation: dreams of particular importance—elevated messages transcending mundane concerns.

### *The Peregrine Condition*

Opposite of essential dignity: the peregrine condition. A planet holding no dignity whatsoever in current position. Latin *peregrinus*: wanderer, stranger. A peregrine planet wanders without authority, like stranger in foreign land. Bonatti: peregrine ninth house ruler indicates false or meaningless dreams. The planetary messenger lacks credentials. Communications cannot be trusted.

Worse: detriment (opposite to domicile) and fall (opposite to exaltation). Ninth house ruler in detriment: dreams actively distorted by planetary discomfort. Ruler in fall: dreams seem significant but prove misleading. Elevated appearances mask hollow content.

### *Combustion and Under the Beams*

A planet approaching conjunction with the Sun enters increasing obscuration. Within 17 degrees: under the beams—light diminished by solar brilliance. Within 8.5 degrees: combust—significations burned up, overwhelmed, hidden. Exception: cazimi. A planet within 17 minutes of exact solar degree is strengthened by heart-of-the-Sun placement.

Combust ninth house ruler: dream's message hidden or overwhelmed. Information exists; dreamer cannot see it clearly. These dreams feel powerful upon waking. Meaning remains out of reach. Do not force interpretation. Wait until planet separates from Sun, or use different method.

## Malefic Affliction

Mars and Saturn—traditional malefics—can afflict the ninth house or its ruler by occupation or hard aspect. Such affliction: dreams arising from fear, anxiety, bodily disturbance rather than prophetic communication. Nightmare produced by Saturn squaring ninth house ruler likely reveals dreamer's anxieties, not future events.

Saturn signals depression, delay, obstruction, fear. In dreams: limitation, imprisonment, failure, death. Most reflect anxiety about worst-case scenarios. A few carry real warnings. To distinguish prophetic warning from projection, examine Saturn's essential dignity and presence or absence of reception.

Mars brings conflict, violence, anger. Hard aspect to ninth house ruler produces vivid dreams of battle, argument, injury. More often reflects bodily heat, repressed anger, recent violent imagery than genuine warning. Mars in its own dignity or received by the planet it afflicts: reliable content.

### *Mitigation Through Reception*

Reception: a planet occupies another planet's domicile. This transforms difficult configurations. Malefic energy integrates rather than destroys. Saturn aspecting ninth house ruler from Capricorn or Aquarius: challenging but instructive dreams. Mars aspecting from Aries or Scorpio: urgent but actionable information.

Mutual reception: two planets each occupy the other's domicile. Strong constructive bond—each bestows strengths on the other. Ninth house ruler in mutual reception with malefic transforms distorting influence into genuine teaching. Dream may contain challenging content; challenge serves prophetic purpose.

## The Moon's Testimony

Moon holds special significance—traditional rulership over night, association with body, emotions, fluctuating states. Moon's condition provides testimony about bodily and emotional factors influencing dream content. Moon afflicted by malefics: dreams arising from physical discomfort. Moon applying to benefics: favorable portent.

Application and separation matter. Applying aspects: developing conditions. Separating aspects: conditions already manifesting or fading. Moon applying to ninth house ruler: dream's message coming into focus. Separating: prophetic moment has passed.

### *Void of Course*

Void-of-course Moon: making no completing aspects before leaving current sign. Traditional doctrine: void Moon questions unreliable or inconsequential. Bonatti extends to dreams: void-of-course Moon at time of dreaming—dream will not produce significant outcomes. Interesting imagery. No prophetic traction. Nothing comes of it.

Exception: Moon void in Cancer (domicile), Taurus (exaltation), or Sagittarius and Pisces (Jupiter's signs, where she holds triplicity dignity). In these signs, Moon retains sufficient essential dignity to signify without completing aspects. Dreams may still carry significance—often internal rather than externally prophetic.

## Synthesis and Judgment

Applying Bonatti's rules requires synthesis, not mechanical addition. Single negative indication does not condemn a dream. Single positive indication does not guarantee prophetic truth. Weigh multiple testimonies. Note which factors dominate. Read overall pattern rather than isolated factors.

Primary test: ninth house ruler's essential dignity. If planet holds domicile, exaltation, or strong triplicity, dream passes first threshold. Ruler peregrine, debilitated, or combust—approach with skepticism regardless of other factors.

*Table 12.4. Ninth House Ruler Conditions and Clinical Actions*

| Ninth House Ruler | Veracity | Clinical Action |
|---|---|---|
| Domicile / Exaltation | High | Proceed to symbolic interpretation |
| Combust (< 8.5° to Sun) | Obscured | Message exists but unreadable; wait |
| Peregrine | Low / None | Treat as psychological noise or somatic |
| Detriment / Fall | Distorted | Proceed with caution; likely misleading |

Secondary tests: malefic affliction, reception, lunar testimony. Dream passing primary but failing secondary may carry genuine content distorted by afflicting factors. Dream passing both deserves serious interpretive attention.

### *The Almuten*

For particularly important dreams, calculate the Almuten of the ninth house cusp—planet exercising greatest combined dignity over that degree. Arabic *al-mubtazz*: the victor. Sum essential dignities each planet holds at that degree. Highest total becomes Almuten. If Almuten also holds favorable accidental conditions—angular, free from combustion, receiving benefic aspects—dream's veracity is strongly supported.

These protocols function as triage. Quick assessment: does this dream warrant serious work? Dreams passing deserve full technique—planetary symbolism, natal chart, timing, narrative content. Dreams failing may reward psychological exploration. They do not require celestial interpretation.

## What Bonatti Teaches

Not all dreams are equal. The art lies in knowing which to trust—and having criteria beyond hope or fear for making that judgment.

Essential dignity is primary. Ninth house ruler's condition provides first assessment. Dignified = reliable. Peregrine = unreliable. This single factor often suffices for initial triage.

Combustion obscures. Combust significator: message exists but cannot be read clearly. Appropriate response is patience, not forced interpretation.

Malefics distort unless received. Saturn and Mars afflicting ninth house or ruler suggest distortion—unless reception transforms configuration. Reception turns destructive energy into instructive challenge.

Moon testifies. Her condition reveals bodily and emotional factors. Void of course: nothing comes of it. Afflicted: physical or emotional disturbance underlies dream.

Synthesis, not mechanism. No single factor determines veracity. Weigh testimonies. Note which dominate. Read pattern. Judgment emerges from integration, not checklist.

## Toward Integration

Preceding chapters traced oneiromancy through historical streams: Mesopotamian omens, Egyptian constitutional types, Vedic validation and timing, Chinese organ-spirit diagnosis, Bön transformational practice, Greek synthesis, Persian-Arabic refinement. This chapter provided Western astrological apparatus: ninth house as locus of prophecy, Bonatti's veracity criteria as method for assessment.

What remains is integration. How do these traditions converge? Where do they diverge? What can contemporary practitioner draw from each? The chapter that follows addresses practical synthesis—navigating between systems, knowing when to apply which framework, building clinical practice that honors multiple lineages while serving the dreamer who sits before you now.

## Sources

Bonatti, Guido. *Liber Astronomiae*. Translated by Benjamin N. Dykes. Minneapolis: Cazimi Press, 2007.

Dorotheus of Sidon. *Carmen Astrologicum*. Translated by David Pingree. Leipzig: Teubner, 1976.

Firmicus Maternus. *Mathesis*. Translated by Jean Rhys Bram. Park Ridge: Noyes Press, 1975.

Lilly, William. *Christian Astrology*. London: 1647. Reprint, Exeter: Regulus, 1985.

Ptolemy. *Tetrabiblos*. Translated by F. E. Robbins. Cambridge: Harvard University Press, 1940.

Valens, Vettius. *Anthology*. Translated by Mark Riley. 2010.

Varāhamihira. *Bṛhat Saṃhitā*. Translated by M. Ramakrishna Bhat. Delhi: Motilal Banarsidass, 1981.

## Chapter Thirteen

# Syncretic Integration

*Πάντα ῥεῖ καὶ οὐδὲν μένει.*

*All things flow and nothing remains.*

—Heraclitus, fr. 91 (Diels-Kranz)

# The Interpreter's Dilemma

The preceding chapters have surveyed eight traditions of dream interpretation, each with its own worldview, method, and remedies. The student now possesses multiple lenses—but multiple lenses can confuse rather than clarify. When a patient presents a dream, which framework should the interpreter apply? The Mesopotamian omen-reader asks what the gods have written. The Egyptian priest assesses the dreamer's constitutional type. The Vedic *daivajña* determines the watch of occurrence and casts a validation chart. The Chinese physician reads organ-spirit imbalance. The Hellenistic *oneirokritēs* classifies the dream's category and weighs contextual factors. The Arabic interpreter considers the dreamer's spiritual state and life-period. The medieval astrologer applies Bonatti's veracity protocols. Which tool, when, how?

Honor each tradition's distinctiveness. Recognize underlying convergences. Different idioms, same sky. Mesopotamian *zaqīqu*, Chinese *hún*, Vedic *svapna*, Greek *oneiros*: same phenomenon, different grammars. Navigate across parallel systems.

# What Each Tradition Contributes

What does each tradition contribute? The following summary distills the core question, method, and clinical utility of each framework examined in this volume.

*Table 13.1 Summary of Dream Perspectives*

| Tradition | Primary Question | Core Method | Clinical Contribution |
|---|---|---|---|
| Non-literate / Oral | What does the community need? | Communal validation and fulfillment | Dreams exist in social context; interpretation is collective responsibility |
| Mesopotamian | What do the gods say? | Omen catalogues + *namburbi* ritual | External message requires ritual response; prognosis enables intervention |

| **Tradition** | **Primary Question** | **Core Method** | **Clinical Contribution** |
|---|---|---|---|
| Egyptian | What type am I? | Constitutional typology (Horian/ Sethian) | Same dream means different things for different constitutions |
| Vedic | When did it occur? Is it valid? | Watch timing + sevenfold classification + validation criteria | Temporal precision + remedial technology (*śānti*) |
| Classical Chinese | What organ is speaking? | Organ-spirit (*wǔ shén*) diagnosis + flavor therapeutics | Dreams as medical symptoms; treatment follows diagnosis |
| Bön (Tibetan) | How can sleep transform? | *Milam* (dream yoga) + chakra-syllable practice | Dreams as bardo rehearsal; death preparation through sleep |
| Hellenistic Greek | What category? What context? | Classification (Macrobius) + context-dependency (Artemidorus) | Not all dreams warrant interpretation; know the dreamer before the dream |
| Persian-Arabic | What life chapter? What spiritual state? | *Firdaria* + threefold classification | Timing by life-period; interpretation participates in manifestation |
| Medieval Latin (Bonatti) | Is this dream true or false? | Essential dignity + lunar testimony | Veracity assessment protocol; not all dreams merit serious attention |

Each tradition contributes something the others lack. Mesopotamian omen-reading provides the principle that dreams can be redirected through timely intervention—what is foreseen need not be suffered. Egyptian constitutional typology recognizes individual variation that renders universal symbol dictionaries unreliable. Vedic temporal analysis provides precision about when a dream will manifest. Classical Chinese organ-spirit diagnosis integrates dream interpretation into comprehensive medical treatment. Bön dream yoga (*milam*) offers techniques for transforming consciousness within the dream itself, using sleep as a vehicle for spiritual realization rather than interpretation. Greek classification prevents the interpreter from wasting effort on somatic noise. Arabic *firdaria* timing situates the dream within the dreamer's life-arc. Bonatti's veracity protocols filter signal from noise. The integrative practitioner draws on all these contributions without collapsing them into homogenized mush.

## The External-Internal Spectrum

Chapter One introduced the concept of an ontological spectrum tracking where traditions locate the dream's origin. This spectrum shows how the traditions relate and why they differ.

At the most external pole stands Mesopotamia, where dreams arrive as messages from deities—communications from outside the dreamer requiring ritual response. The dream-god Zaqīqu blows divine messages into the passive sleeper like wind. The dreamer is a receiver, not a generator. Interpretation serves state prognostication; personal meaning is secondary to collective portent.

Moving inward, Egyptian oneiromancy occupies a threshold position. The dream (*resut*) is understood as an awakening into liminal space where external divine communication meets internal constitutional reception. The Horian/Sethian typology recognizes that the same external message registers differently depending on the dreamer's inherent nature. The Four Sons of Horus map received influence on specific internal organs. Egypt begins the internalization process that will reach completion in China.

Indian and Greek traditions represent intermediate positions where divine, celestial, and somatic factors coexist without systematic hierarchy. The Vedic tradition views the dream as a messenger of the gods (*dūta*) while acknowledging that humoral imbalances (*doṣas*) can generate imagery. Greek development, particularly under Artemidorus and Macrobius, distinguishes prophetic visions from meaningless nocturnal disturbances arising from bodily states. Both traditions preserve the external possibility while making room for internal causation.

At the most internal pole, Classical Chinese Medicine represents the fully internalized model. Dreams arise from the condition of the five organ-spirits, with the ethereal soul (*hún*) of the Liver bearing primary responsibility for dream activity. The sky has been fully internalized; the Eight Extraordinary Vessels serve as internal wiring for celestial influences. Dream diagnosis reads the movement of spirit through the organ systems as physiological feedback rather than an external omen. The gods have become organs; prophecy has become diagnosis.

The Bön tradition of Zhang Zhung occupies a unique position after the Chinese internalization. Rather than reading dreams as external messages or internal symptoms, Bön *milam* (dream yoga) treats the dream as a transformational field. The four daytime foundations (changing karmic traces, removing grasping and aversion, strengthening intention, cultivating memory) and four nighttime phases (throat/peace, brow/clarity, heart/presence, secret/fearlessness) constitute a technology for working within the dream state itself. The seed syllables *A, OM, HUNG,* correlated with chakras and elements, provide anchors for maintaining awareness through the dissolution that sleep brings. Where Chinese medicine diagnoses, Bön transforms. Where other traditions interpret what dreams mean, Bön trains practitioners to transform while dreaming—and explicitly frames this as rehearsal for the *bardo* states encountered at death. The dreamer is neither a passive receiver nor a diagnostic subject but an active participant in consciousness transformation. From here, the Western traditions—Greek, Persian-Arabic, Medieval Latin—develop their own syntheses.

*Table 13.2 Comparative Framework Across Traditions*

| Tradition | Dream Source | Interpretation Mode | Remediation Focus |
|---|---|---|---|
| Mesopotamian | External (Zaqīqu / Deities) | Ominal (Prognosis of state/fate) | Apotropaic ritual (*namburbi*) |
| Egyptian | Threshold (Liminal) | Constitutional typology | Ritual and organ attention |
| Vedic | Celestial-Karmic | *Doṣa* and *guṇa* mediated | Timing and propitiation |
| Classical Chinese | Internal (*hún / pò*) | *Zàng-fŭ* diagnostic feedback | Medical and flavor intervention |
| Bön (Tibetan) | Transformational (*rigpa* / awareness) | Chakra-syllable visualization + *milam* | Dream yoga and bardo preparation |
| Greek | Divine/Somatic mixed | Context-dependent classification | Incubation and medicine |

The spectrum determines intervention. An externally-sourced dream requires ritual response—propitiation, protection, redirection of fate. An internally-sourced dream requires medical response—herbs, acupuncture, lifestyle modification, dietary adjustment. A threshold dream may require both. First question: where on this spectrum does the dream fall?

# Convergences Across Traditions

Despite their different ontologies and methods, the traditions examined in this volume converge on several fundamental principles. These convergences are cross-cultural wisdom. Different civilizations, same phenomenon, same conclusions.

## *Classification Precedes Interpretation*

Every tradition distinguishes meaningful dreams from noise. Macrobius offers his fivefold classification; the Vedic system its sevenfold. Artemidorus separates *enhypnia* (somatic dreams) from *oneiroi* (prophetic dreams). The *Suśruta Saṃhitā* isolates the *bhāvika* (prophetic) type from six others lacking predictive weight. Classical

Chinese Medicine recognizes that dreams of excess differ from dreams of deficiency. Bonatti provides protocols for determining veracity before interpretation begins. The convergence is universal: not all dreams deserve serious attention, and determining which do is the interpreter's first task.

## *Timing Matters*

The Vedic system divides the night into four watches, each with a different manifestation range. The Arabic tradition uses *firdaria* to situate dreams within life-periods. Chapter Three introduced the tripartite night governed by triplicity lords. The Achuar *hora de wayusa* at 3–4 AM corresponds precisely to the Vedic fourth watch when dreams most reliably come true. Across traditions, the way a dream occurs affects its meaning and predictive weight. The interpreter must ask: what time did you wake from this dream?

## *Context and Constitution Shape Meaning*

Egyptian constitutional typology recognizes that the same symbol means different things for Horians and Sethians. Artemidorus insists that the interpreter must know the dreamer's profession, social status, health, and circumstances before interpreting symbols. Ibn Sīrīn teaches that the same dream carries a different weight for a righteous person and an unrighteous one. Classical Chinese Medicine reads identical dream content differently depending on the patient's underlying pattern. Universal symbol dictionaries fail because symbols are not universal; they are filtered through the individual's constitution, culture, and current circumstances.

## *Dreams Can Be Redirected*

The Mesopotamian *namburbi* rituals demonstrate that adverse dreams need not manifest. Vedic tradition prescribes *śānti* (pacification) rituals and specific mantras for dream neutralization. Classical Chinese Medicine treats the underlying organ imbalance to resolve the dream pattern. Even Bonatti's veracity protocols serve a remedial function: knowing a dream is false frees the dreamer from anxiety. The traditions converge on the principle that prognosis enables intervention. What is foreseen can be redirected; what is diagnosed can be treated. Fatalism contradicts the purpose of interpretation.

### *The Interpreter Participates in Manifestation*

Ibn Sīrīn teaches that the dream is on the wing of a bird until interpreted—meaning its significance remains malleable until spoken. The Haudenosaunee *Ononharoia* demonstrates that communal interpretation fulfills the soul's hidden wish, thereby averting illness. The interpreter's framing participates in what the dream becomes. This places ethical weight on the act of interpretation: to speak carelessly is to shape destiny carelessly. The traditions converge in recognizing that interpretation is not passive reception but active participation.

## Divergences Among Traditions

The convergences should not obscure genuine disagreements. These divergences are not merely terminological; they reflect fundamentally different understandings of what dreams are and what purpose interpretation serves.

### *External Message versus Internal Diagnosis*

Mesopotamian oneiromancy treats the dream as divine communication requiring ritual response. Classical Chinese Medicine treats the dream as physiological feedback requiring medical intervention. These are incompatible ontologies. A practitioner cannot simultaneously believe the dream is a message from Zaqīqu and a symptom of Liver Blood deficiency. The integrative practitioner must recognize when external-message interpretation serves the patient and when internal-diagnostic interpretation serves better—without claiming both are really the same thing.

### *Fixed Symbols versus Contextual Meaning*

Mesopotamian dream books operate through fixed correspondences: dreaming of a raven (*āribu*) portends income increase (*irbu*) because the words sound similar. Artemidorus explicitly rejects this approach, insisting that symbols must be interpreted in context. The same dream of plowing a field means one thing for a farmer (work ahead), another for a merchant (profit from labor), another for a bachelor (marriage). Chinese organ-spirit diagnosis occupies a middle position: there are standard correspondences (fire dreams indicate Heart disturbance), but they must be contextualized within the patient's overall pattern. The interpreter must decide whether to apply dictionary lookup or contextual analysis.

### *Prophetic Focus versus Diagnostic Focus*

Western traditions—Mesopotamian, Greek, Arabic, Medieval Latin—primarily concern themselves with prophecy: what will happen? Classical Chinese Medicine primarily concerns itself with diagnosis: what is happening internally? These different orientations produce different interpretive methods. Prophetic interpretation asks whether the dream is true and when it will manifest. Diagnostic interpretation asks which organ system is disturbed and what treatment is indicated. A dream can be interpreted both ways, but the interpreter must recognize which question is being answered.

### *Individual versus Communal Interpretation*

Western, Greek, and Islamic traditions emphasize the expert interpreter who decodes symbols for the individual dreamer. Aboriginal, Haudenosaunee, and Achuar traditions treat dreaming as communal property requiring collective interpretation. In oral traditions, the dream belongs to the community; its fulfillment is a collective responsibility. The solo practitioner working with an individual patient operates in a different social frame than the Sangoma whose interpretation carries weight for the entire village. The integrative practitioner in contemporary Western settings cannot simply import communal protocols, but can recognize when a patient's dream concerns not only their individual welfare but their place within family, community, or society.

## Clinical Navigation: When to Apply Which Framework

Convergences and divergences yield decision criteria. What follows is not an algorithm but a heuristic.

### *First Question: Is This Dream Worth Interpreting?*

Apply Macrobius's fivefold classification and Bonatti's veracity protocols. If the dream appears to be *insomnium* (nightmare from bodily disturbance) or *visum* (hypnagogic apparition), medical assessment may be indicated, but prophetic interpretation is not. If Bonatti's criteria show the ninth lord peregrine or combust, or the Moon void of course, the dream likely carries no portent. This first filter prevents the interpreter from wasting effort and the patient from receiving false significance.

## *Second Question: When Did It Occur?*

Apply Vedic watch-timing. Dreams in the first watch (sunset to approximately 10 PM) carry long manifestation ranges and mixed reliability; dreams in the fourth watch (3 AM to sunrise) carry short manifestation ranges and high reliability. If the patient reports the dream occurring just before dawn and not returning to sleep afterward, take the dream more seriously. If the dream occurred in the first watch after heavy eating, consider somatic causation.

## *Third Question: What Is the Patient's Constitution and Current State?*

Apply Egyptian constitutional assessment and Chinese pattern diagnosis. Is this a Horian type (stable, tradition-bound) or a Sethian type (chaotic, boundary-crossing)? What is the underlying pattern—excess or deficiency, heat or cold, internal or external? What is the patient's current life circumstance? Symbols must be interpreted through this constitutional filter. A dream of fire means something different for a patient with Heart fire excess than for a patient with Kidney yang deficiency.

## *Fourth Question: What Life-Period Is the Patient In?*

Apply *firdaria* or a similar chronocrator. A dream during Saturn's period carries a different weight than the same dream during Jupiter's period. Dreams during the twelfth-house profection year concern confinement, isolation, and dissolution. Dreams during the ninth-house profection year concern meaning, travel, and higher knowledge. The same symbol acquires different significance depending on where in the life cycle it appears.

### *Fifth Question: Is This Dream Calling for Ritual or Medicine?*

Apply the external-internal spectrum. If the dream appears to carry external portent—warning of events in the world, visitation by figures who feel non-personal—consider ritual response: prayer, protective rites, or the equivalent of *namburbi*. If the dream appears to reflect internal process—bodily symptoms, emotional processing, organ-spirit communication—consider medical response: herbs, acupuncture, dietary modification, lifestyle adjustment. Many dreams call for both.

#### *Sixth Question: What Does the Dream Content Suggest?*

Only after these contextual questions have been addressed should the interpreter turn to symbol analysis. Apply Chinese organ-spirit correspondences (fire = Heart, water = Kidney, anger = Liver) alongside Artemidoran contextual interpretation. Does the dream involve recurring themes that suggest alchemical stage-work? Does the imagery point toward specific planetary influences that can be verified against current transits? Symbol interpretation is the last step, not the first, because symbols without context are ambiguous.

## Modern Analytical Methods

Modern psychological approaches developed in dialogue with these traditions. Brief orientation follows. .

### *Depth Psychology*

Freud's *Traumdeutung* (1899) established the modern psychological study of dreams, distinguishing manifest content (the dream as remembered) from latent content (the underlying wish). Dream-work transforms latent content through condensation, displacement, and symbolization. While Freud's specific theories of wish-fulfillment and sexual symbolism remain contested, his fundamental insight—that dreams require interpretation rather than literal reading—aligns with Artemidorus's distinction between theorematic (literal) and allegorical dreams.

Jung expanded dream interpretation beyond personal psychology to include archetypal and collective dimensions. The collective unconscious contains primordial images (archetypes) that appear in dreams across cultures. Jung's method of amplification—connecting dream images to mythological, religious, and cultural parallels—resembles the comparative approach employed throughout this volume. Active imagination, where the dreamer continues dialogue with dream figures in waking consciousness, provides a contemporary parallel to incubation practices.

## *Gestalt Approach*

Fritz Perls proposed that every element of the dream represents an aspect of the dreamer. The method involves the dreamer speaking as each dream element, discovering through role-play what that element expresses. This radically internal approach contrasts with external-message traditions but complements Chinese organ-spirit diagnosis: if the fire in the dream is an aspect of the dreamer, it may be the Heart-fire speaking.

## *Phenomenological Approaches*

Medard Boss's *Daseinsanalysis* approaches dreams as revelations of being-in-the-world rather than as symbolic codes requiring translation. The dream discloses how the dreamer exists; interpretation attends to what is present rather than searching for hidden meaning. This approach resembles the Egyptian understanding of *resut* as awakening—the dream reveals what is already there.

## *Neuroscientific Frameworks*

Contemporary sleep science distinguishes REM and non-REM sleep, maps neural activation patterns during dreaming, and proposes functional theories including memory consolidation and threat simulation. The activation-synthesis hypothesis suggests that dreams are the forebrain's attempt to make sense of random brainstem signals—a view incompatible with prophetic interpretation but potentially compatible with somatic-noise filtering. The integrative practitioner need not resolve scientific debates but should recognize that REM rebound (intensified dreaming after suppression from alcohol or medication) produces dreams that may reflect physiology rather than prophecy.

# Alchemical Dreamwork

Western alchemy reads dreams as stages of soul-transformation. The alchemical *opus*—transforming base metal into gold—mirrors the psyche's work of integrating unconscious contents into conscious wholeness. Dreams mark progress through this work, and the skilled interpreter learns to recognize which stage the dreamer currently inhabits. The celestial framework provides diagnostic precision: planetary transits and periods trigger specific stages, natal configurations predispose to prolonged work at particular phases, and the dream chart itself reveals which alchemical operation the dream performs.

Paracelsus identified three fundamental principles: *Sal* (Salt, body, fixed matter), *Mercurius* (Mercury, spirit, volatile principle), and *Sulphur* (Sulfur, soul, combustible essence). Salt dreams concern the body—physical symptoms, material circumstances, concrete imagery. Mercury dreams concern spirit—communication, movement, trickery, shapeshifting, paradox. Sulfur dreams concern soul—passion, desire, burning, conflict, sexuality, creative fire. When a dream resists interpretation, asking whether this is Salt, Mercury, or Sulfur often clarifies which dimension of the dreamer's life the dream addresses.

Process unfolds through four color-stages, each governed by a planetary principle and marked by characteristic dream imagery.

## *Nigredo (Blackening)*

Saturn's stage. Dreams of death, decay, descent, corpses, ravens, black earth, dismemberment. Old self dies. These dreams feel like failure but signal that transformation has begun. The dreamer may wake in dread, convinced that something is terribly wrong. The alchemical interpreter recognizes *nigredo* dreams as necessary dissolution—the *putrefactio* that precedes new growth. Without the rotting of the seed, no sprout emerges. Clinically, *nigredo* dreams often accompany life transitions: divorce, job loss, serious illness, the death of someone close. The interpreter's task is to reframe apparent catastrophe as initiation.

*Nigredo* correlates with Saturn transits to natal Sun, Moon, or Ascendant; Saturn's station on a sensitive degree; or the onset of *Śani mahādaśā*. In the dream chart, Saturn, angular or ruling the ninth house, marks the dream as *nigredo* material. Natives with natal Saturn in the twelfth, eighth, or conjunct the Moon may experience prolonged *nigredo* phases requiring particular attention to prevent fixation in the blackening. Saturn's return (approximately ages 29, 58, 87) frequently initiates fresh *nigredo* work.

The iconography of the *Rosarium Philosophorum* (1550) depicts *nigredo* as the king and queen naked, stripped of pretense, sinking into the mercurial bath. Saturn's traditional association with death, time, and limitation governs this stage; the *Mutus Liber* shows the blackening under Saturn's seal. George Ripley's *Compound of Alchemy* (1471) describes the *nigredo* as the "black of blacks, blacker than black"—the complete absence of light that precedes its return.

## Albedo (Whitening)

Moon's stage. Dreams of washing, purification, snow, silver, dawn, white birds, clear water, bathing. The *nigredo*'s blackness washes clean. Feminine principle emerges; emotion clarifies. Dreams shift from death imagery to cleansing imagery. The dreamer may encounter feminine figures—mother, sister, unknown woman, goddess—who guide or instruct. Luna presides; receptivity replaces resistance. The interpreter watches for premature solar assertion that would abort the whitening process. *Albedo* requires patience, reflection, and the courage to not-know.

*Albedo* correlates with lunar progressions, secondary progressed Moon to sensitive degrees, or Moon *daśā*. Transiting Jupiter's trine or sextile to natal Moon may support the whitening process; harsh Saturn aspects may delay it. Natives with strong Moon-Neptune configurations experience deep *albedo* work, sometimes extending over years. Prolonged water element emphasis in transits (outer planets through water signs aspecting the natal chart) sustains the purification phase.

Michael Maier's *Atalanta Fugiens* (1617) depicts the Moon governing this phase, her silver light washing away Saturn's darkness. The association of the Moon with purification, reflection, and the feminine appears consistently across alchemical sources. The interpreter watches for premature solar assertion that would abort the whitening process. When a dreamer in *albedo* asks what they should do, the correct answer is often: wait, listen, let the water do its work. The temptation to rush toward clarity (*citrinitas*) before purification completes produces incomplete transformation.

## *Citrinitas (Yellowing)*

Sun's stage. Dreams of sunrise, gold appearing, dawning light, yellow flowers, awakening after a long sleep. Solar consciousness rises. Some alchemists collapsed this stage into *rubedo*, but where the stage is distinguished, it marks the emergence of insight: the dreamer sees clearly what was previously obscure. Dreams may feature illumination, discovery, finding treasure, solving puzzles, teachers who explain, and light breaking through clouds.

*Citrinitas* correlates with solar arcs to natal positions, progressed Sun aspects, or Sun *daśā*. Jupiter transits to the natal Sun or crossing angular cusps support the emergence of clarity. The yellowing marks the transition from lunar receptivity to solar understanding. What was received in *albedo* now becomes conscious understanding in *citrinitas*. Bonus of Ferrara's *Margarita Pretiosa* describes the yellowing as the appearance of the golden head that signals approaching completion.

Clinically, *citrinitas* dreams signal that the patient can now articulate what they have been going through. The naming that was impossible during *nigredo* and premature during *albedo* becomes possible. The interpreter supports this emergence of clarity without rushing toward integration before the insight fully crystallizes.

## *Rubedo (Reddening)*

Integration. Dreams of the red king and white queen united, *coniunctio oppositorum*, phoenix rising from ashes, blood that heals rather than wounds. Self manifests. Opposites that warred through earlier stages now marry. Dreams of union, wedding, birth, completion, red and white together, sun and moon conjoined. The *lapis philosophorum* (philosopher's stone) emerges—not external gold but internal wholeness. The interpreter recognizes *rubedo* dreams as signals that a cycle of transformation nears completion. The dreamer is ready to return to ordinary life, carrying new capacity.

*Rubedo* correlates with Jupiter-Venus conjunctions, mutual receptions between benefics, or benefic transits to the natal Sun-Moon midpoint. Mars properly integrated (trine or sextile from benefics) provides the red sulfuric fire without destructive combustion. Natives with T-squares or grand crosses face more difficult *rubedo* work, but the integration they achieve proves more comprehensive; oppositions resolved become the strongest structures.

Yet *rubedo* is not an ending—it is a plateau from which new *nigredo* may begin. The spiral continues; the *opus* renews; the stone must be made again at deeper levels. The interpreter who recognizes completed *rubedo* can release the dreamer into life, trusting that dreams will call them back when the next blackening begins.

### *The Spiral Path*

These stages do not proceed linearly. A dreamer may cycle through *nigredo* multiple times, or regress from *albedo* to *nigredo* when a new layer of unconscious material surfaces. Saturn returns every twenty-nine years; each return may initiate fresh *nigredo*. The stages describe a spiral rather than a ladder—each revolution passes through the same colors at greater depth.

The interpreter tracks where the dreamer stands, recognizes which work the current dream performs, and resists the temptation to rush the process. A dreamer deep in *nigredo* cannot be counseled into *citrinitas*; the blackening must complete. A dreamer lingering in *albedo* may need gentle encouragement toward the solar emergence they fear. Celestial timing anchors the framework: where the dreamer stands, how long the phase lasts—Saturn transits have known duration; *daśā* periods have calculated extent. This temporal knowledge transforms interpretation from guess into guidance.

## Worked Examples

Theory requires demonstration. Two examples of dreams interpreted through multiple frameworks, showing how the integrative practitioner navigates between systems. The dreams are composites drawn from clinical experience; no actual patient is represented.

## *Example One: The Collapsing House*

A forty-five-year-old woman reports a recurring dream in which the house she lived in as a child begins collapsing around her. She runs from room to room trying to save precious objects, but the floors keep giving way. She woke at approximately 4:30 AM from the most recent occurrence, breathing rapidly, unable to return to sleep.

*Veracity assessment*: The dream occurred in the fourth watch, suggesting high reliability if prophetic. Saturn currently transits her natal Moon. The ninth house of her nativity contains Saturn; at the time of the dream, Saturn ruled the hour. These factors suggest a dream worth serious attention.

*Chinese organ-spirit diagnosis*: Dreams of buildings collapsing correlate with Spleen deficiency (the Spleen governs the flesh and the sense of solidity, of being held up). Dreams of running without reaching safety suggest Liver constraint (the *hún* is unable to find rest). The patient confirms chronic digestive complaints and a tendency to rumination.

*Alchemical staging*: The collapsing structure, the inability to preserve what matters, the sense that ground itself cannot be trusted—these are *nigredo* markers. Saturn transiting the natal Moon confirms the timing. The woman is midlife, entering her second Saturn opposition. Old structures that seemed permanent are revealing their impermanence.

*Constitutional assessment*: The patient presents as Horian (stable, tradition-bound, valuing the familiar). The dream's Sethian imagery—chaos, dissolution, boundary-collapse—represents what her constitution most fears. The dream confronts her with what she has excluded.

*Integrative response*: The practitioner addresses the Spleen deficiency medically (digestive support, dietary modification). The practitioner frames the dream as *nigredo* initiation rather than catastrophe, normalizing the Saturn transit and providing temporal context (the transit will pass within months). The practitioner does not offer premature reassurance—the house that must fall must fall—but provides the frame that allows falling to become transformation rather than mere destruction.

## *Example Two: The Luminous Stranger*

A thirty-two-year-old man reports a dream in which a figure made of golden light appeared in his bedroom, communicated wordlessly that he would receive guidance, and left through the window, ascending into the sky. He woke feeling profound peace at approximately 5:15 AM. He had eaten lightly the evening before and had no alcohol.

*Veracity assessment*: Fourth watch, just before sunrise—maximum reliability. The patient did not return to sleep. Jupiter currently trines his natal Sun. The Moon was applying to Jupiter at the time of waking. These factors suggest a *visio* (prophetic vision) or *oraculum* (oracular communication) rather than *insomnium* or *visum*.

*Chinese organ-spirit diagnosis*: Luminous imagery, ascent, a sense of communication without words—these suggest *shén* (Heart-spirit) activity. The peaceful affect upon waking indicates the *shén* is settled; this is not a dream of pathology but of spiritual opening.

*Alchemical staging*: The golden light, the communication of guidance, the sense of completion—these suggest *citrinitas* or early *rubedo*. Jupiter's trine to the natal Sun supports this assessment. Something the patient has been working toward is beginning to integrate.

*Constitutional assessment*: The patient presents as a mixed type with Sethian tendencies (creative, boundary-pushing, drawn to the unusual). The luminous stranger represents the ordering principle his constitution typically resists. The dream brings complementary energy.

*Integrative response*: The practitioner receives the dream as authentic communication, not requiring medical intervention. The practitioner encourages the patient to attend to what guidance may come in the following days (the dream announces guidance but does not deliver it). The practitioner notes the Jupiter transit and frames the current period as propitious for decisions the patient may have been delaying. No ritual response is necessary; the dream itself is the blessing.

# Toward the Botanical Allies

The traditions examined in this volume share not only interpretive methods but remedial technologies. Among these, the use of plant allies to facilitate dream access, enhance dream recall, and anchor dream guidance holds particular importance. The Sangoma's *ubulawu* preparation, the Achuar's guayusa (*Ilex guayusa*) tea, and the widespread use of mugwort (*Artemisia vulgaris*) across European and Asian traditions all represent the intersection of herbalism with oneiromancy.

The chapter that follows addresses the botanical dimension: plants that open the dream gate, plants that clarify dream content, plants that preserve dream memory into waking, and plants that anchor the dreamer against the disorientation that vivid dreaming can produce. These allies have their own planetary signatures, their own organ affinities, their own contraindications and cautions. Their integration with celestial timing allows the practitioner to select the appropriate ally for the patient's constitution, current planetary period, and interpretive need.

What remains after the botanical chapter is practice itself. The technologies surveyed in this volume—celestial, medical, psychological, botanical—serve the moment when a patient sits before the interpreter and says: I had a dream. Everything converges toward that moment. May the interpreter be equal to what it requires.

# Sources

Abū Ma'shar. *Kitāb al-Mudkhal al-Kabīr*. Translated by Charles Burnett. *The Great Introduction to Astrology*. 2 vols. Leiden: Brill, 2019.

Artemidorus. *Oneirocritica*. Translated by Robert J. White. *The Interpretation of Dreams*. Park Ridge, NJ: Noyes Press, 1975.

Bonatti, Guido. *Liber Astronomiae*. Translated by Benjamin N. Dykes. *Book of Astronomy*. Golden Valley, MN: Cazimi Press, 2007.

Boss, Medard. *The Analysis of Dreams*. London: Rider, 1957.

Bulkeley, Kelly. *Dreaming in the World's Religions: A Comparative History*. New York: New York University Press, 2008.

Chögyal Namkhai Norbu. *Dream Yoga and the Practice of Natural Light.* Edited by Michael Katz. Ithaca: Snow Lion Publications, 1992.

Dodds, E. R. *The Greeks and the Irrational.* Berkeley: University of California Press, 1951.

Freud, Sigmund. *Die Traumdeutung.* Leipzig: Franz Deuticke, 1899. Translated by James Strachey as *The Interpretation of Dreams.* New York: Basic Books, 1955.

Ibn Sīrīn, Muḥammad. *Tafsīr al-Aḥlām.* Translated as *Dreams and Interpretations.* London: Dar Al-Taqwa, 2000.

Jung, C. G. *Dreams.* Translated by R. F. C. Hull. Princeton: Princeton University Press, 1974.

Jung, C. G. *Psychology and Alchemy.* Translated by R. F. C. Hull. Princeton: Princeton University Press, 1968.

Maciocia, Giovanni. *The Psyche in Chinese Medicine: Treatment of Emotional and Mental Disharmonies with Acupuncture and Chinese Herbs.* Edinburgh: Churchill Livingstone, 2009.

Macrobius. *Commentarii in Somnium Scipionis.* Translated by William Harris Stahl. *Commentary on the Dream of Scipio.* New York: Columbia University Press, 1952.

Maier, Michael. *Atalanta Fugiens.* Oppenheim: Johann Theodor de Bry, 1617. Facsimile edition with translation by Joscelyn Godwin. Grand Rapids: Phanes Press, 1989.

Oberhelman, Steven M. *Dreambooks in Byzantium: Six Oneirocritica in Translation.* Aldershot: Ashgate, 2008.

Oppenheim, A. Leo. *The Interpretation of Dreams in the Ancient Near East.* Transactions of the American Philosophical Society 46.3. Philadelphia: American Philosophical Society, 1956.

Perls, Fritz. *Gestalt Therapy Verbatim.* Lafayette, CA: Real People Press, 1969.

Ripley, George. *The Compound of Alchemy.* London: Thomas Orwin, 1591. Facsimile in *Theatrum Chemicum Britannicum,* edited by Elias Ashmole. London, 1652.

Rochberg, Francesca. *The Heavenly Writing: Divination, Horoscopy, and Astronomy in Mesopotamian Culture.* Cambridge: Cambridge University Press, 2004.

Shulman, David, and Guy G. Stroumsa, eds. *Dream Cultures: Explorations in the Comparative History of Dreaming*. Oxford: Oxford University Press, 1999.

Suśruta. *Suśruta Saṃhitā*. Translated by Kaviraj Kunja Lal Bhishagratna. 3 vols. Calcutta: Bose, 1907–1916.

Tedlock, Barbara, ed. *Dreaming: Anthropological and Psychological Interpretations*. Cambridge: Cambridge University Press, 1987.

Tenzin Wangyal Rinpoche. *The Tibetan Yogas of Dream and Sleep*. Ithaca: Snow Lion Publications, 1998.

Varāhamihira. *Bṛhat Saṃhitā*. Translated by M. Ramakrishna Bhat. 2 vols. Delhi: Motilal Banarsidass, 1981–1982.

## Chapter Fourteen

# Oneirobotany

*šammu ša šamê šubatšu*

*The plant whose home is heaven*

—Babylonian pharmacological formula

# Plant Allies of the Dreaming Soul

Certain plants open the gates of sleep. Others clarify what passes through. Still others ensure the dreamer returns with the message intact.

These are oneirogens — from Greek óneiros (dream) and -gen (producing). They facilitate dream access without overwhelming waking consciousness. They work with the natural architecture of sleep rather than displacing it.

Three functions organize the materia medica that follows. **Opening**: rendering the threshold permeable so the dreamer who previously slept without dreams begins to dream. **Clarifying**: sharpening prophetic capacity so the dreamer receives specific guidance rather than diffuse imagery. **Preserving**: strengthening recall so the dreamer wakes with the message intact rather than watching it dissolve in morning light. Some plants accomplish more than one function. Selection depends on what the patient needs.

Traditions examined here span four thousand years: cuneiform tablets from Nineveh; temple incubation in classical Greece; ubulawu practices of southern African diviners; medhya rasāyana of Āyurveda. These are coherent disciplines — developed through millennia of observation, refined through ritual application, preserved in written records and living transmission.

Each major oneirogen carries a planetary signature guiding selection. Moon for general opening. Mercury for recall and clarity. Jupiter for prophetic vision. Saturn for ancestral communion. Venus for receptive states. The practitioner does not prescribe "a dream herb" but selects a precise ally whose celestial alignment addresses the diagnostic picture.

# Mesopotamian Foundations

Mesopotamia developed the most systematic dream culture of the ancient world. At its center stood the Mesopotamia developed the most systematic dream culture of the ancient world. At its center stood the *Iškar Zaqīqu*, a canonical series of eleven tablets recovered from Ashurbanipal's library at Nineveh. Nine tablets catalogue dream omens with their interpretations; two prescribe ritual remedies for averting evil dreams. The series takes its name from the god Zaqīqu, whose domain was precisely this phenomenon — the *zaqīqu*, the wind-like aspect of the self that departs the body during sleep and travels through other realms, returning with knowledge the waking mind could not otherwise reach.

Evidence begins in the Early Dynastic period (ca. 2500–2340 BCE). By Old Babylonian times the practice had refined into standardized series — approximately one thousand medical tablets at Nineveh. Four types of dreams were recognized: message dreams in which a deity speaks directly; symbolic dreams requiring interpretation; omen dreams predicting future events; and symptomatic dreams reflecting the dreamer's ritual purity or contamination. Good dreams indicated divine favor. Bad dreams signaled demonic interference, witchcraft, or spiritual pollution.

## The Practitioners

Dream diviners came from the highest ranks of Mesopotamian scholarship. The Questioner (*šā›ilu*) might be Exorcist (*āšipu*), Seer (*bārû*), or ecstatic prophet. At the court of Mari, prophetic letters recorded divine messages received through dreams — matters from temple maintenance to military intelligence.

Dream management required collaboration. The Therapeutic Physician (*asû*) treated physical symptoms. The Exorcist (*āšipu*) addressed spiritual causes — divine wrath, demonic influence. In oneirobotany these roles proved inseparable. A dream could reflect physical health or constitute a divine message. The goddess Gula, patroness of medicine, bridged both worlds.

## The Ritual Apparatus

Dream rituals employed consistent elements. Fumigation with sacred plants created atmospheric conditions for divine contact — smoke carrying prayers upward, suffusing the sleeper's environment with protection and vision. The *kukru*-plant, sulphur, and salt appear prominently among fumigants, purifying space and person simultaneously.

Incantations addressed Šamaš, the sun god, alongside the dreamer's personal deity and the gods Ea and Marduk. The Marduk-Ea incantation — documented across nearly three millennia of continuous use — follows a six-part structure: the affliction is described; Marduk becomes aware and consults Ea, who responds with the formula "What I know, you know"; the remedy is transmitted; and the ritual solution enacted. By reciting this divine dialogue, the practitioner positioned the dreamer within a cosmic conversation already underway — one in which the cure had, in a sense, already been given.

## *The Pharmacopoeia*

The *Uruanna* lexicon contains approximately 1,300 terms describing some 340 plants. To induce mantic dreams, practitioners employed mandrake (*Mandragora officinarum*) for its sedative and hallucinogenic properties; cannabis (*Cannabis sativa*) and opium poppy (*Papaver somniferum*) for deep sleep; and darnel (*Lolium temulentum*) — a neurotoxin in controlled doses — to induce states interpreted as divine presence. Beer served as the common carrier. Aromatics including cedar (*Cedrus libani*), myrtle (*Myrtus communis*), and asafoetida (*Ferula assa-foetida*) were burned in censers during incubation.

## *Incubation and Apotropaia*

Two ritual objectives governed practice: *incubation*, which solicited favorable dreams, and *apotropaia*, which nullified unfavorable ones.

Incubation invited the deity or Dream-Spirit (*zaqīqu*) to deliver a message through ritual hygiene, formal prayer to Šamaš, arrangement of censers with specific woods, prescribed physical postures, cleansing baths, offerings, and divine images sketched near the sleeper's bed.

Interpretation followed deductive logic preserved in the eleven tablets, employing linguistic puns that revealed the deep structure of reality. When a dream was bad, apotropaic rituals averted consequences through symbolic transfer, ritual bathing, and aromatic fumigation. The *kurbannu* (clod incantation) transferred dream evil to a ritually prepared substitute — earth molded into human form, receiving the nightmare's malevolence, then destroyed or buried.

Similar substitution rituals used figurines absorbing demonic forces responsible for disturbing dreams, then burned or thrown into flowing water.

Timing mattered. The month of Abu (July/August) marked the period when spirits traveled between netherworld and living world, making protective rituals especially potent — and especially necessary. Dawn rituals invoked Nusku, the protective night light, before greeting Šamaš as the sun rose: night's passage from vulnerability to restored safety.

## Integration with Celestial Medicine

Mesopotamian dream practice operated within a cosmology that read the heavens as divine inscription — celestial events encoding divine intention in patterns legible to trained observers. Dreams represented another surface on which this writing appeared. The *zaqīqu* traveled through the same cosmos that astrologers mapped, and its experiences during sleep reflected the same divine communications that stars and planets encoded.

The plant *maštakal* — whose home is heaven — belongs to this understanding. Substances facilitating dream contact possessed celestial origin or correspondence. The boundary between pharmacology and astrology, between plant and planet, remained permeable. What opened the channel to divine dreams was always, in some sense, heaven reaching down.

## Transcultural Traditions

### *Mediterranean*

Asclepian temple incubation likely incorporated plant allies. Egyptian practice made explicit use of blue lotus (*Nymphaea caerulea*) — the flower appears ubiquitously in temple art and funerary scenes depicting altered states. European traditions center on mugwort (*Artemisia vulgaris*), supplemented by rosemary (*Salvia rosmarinus*), bay laurel (*Laurus nobilis*), and lavender (*Lavandula angustifolia*).

## *African Ubulawu*

Among the Xhosa and Zulu, *ubulawu* refers to dream-inducing preparations used by diviners (*sangoma*) for ancestral communication. The primary plant is African dream root (*Silene capensis*), known in Xhosa as *undlela ziimhlophe* ("white paths") — vivid dreams understood as ancestral messages. Structure parallels Mesopotamian practice: plant as bridge, practitioner with specific intention, dreams as meaningful communications.

## *Mesoamerican*

Among the Chontal Maya, dream herb (*Calea zacatechichi*), called *thle-pelakano* ("leaf of god"), serves for divinatory dreaming — obtaining answers to specific questions through prophetic vision. Research confirms increased dream recall and vividness. Mechanism unknown.

## *Āyurvedic*

Āyurveda contributes *medhya rasāyana* — intellect-rejuvenating substances enhancing cognitive function including dream recall and clarity. Chief among these is intellect tree (*Celastrus paniculatus*), called *jyotiṣmatī* ("the luminous one"). Where other oneirogens open gates or intensify vision, *jyotiṣmatī* ensures the dreamer returns with the message intact.

## *Classical Chinese Medicine*

Classical Chinese Medicine approaches oneirobotany through the Five Spirits (*wǔ shén*) framework, addressing physiological substrate rather than directly inducing oneiric states. Sour jujube seed (*suān zǎo rén*) nourishes Heart Blood and calms the *shén*, providing a material basis for stable *hún* travel. The approach treats root conditions producing disordered dreaming — deficiency rather than absence — restoring substrate before stimulating oneirogens can open gates.

# Materia Medica

## *Purification and Ritual Cleansing*

**Heavenly Plant (Prickly Saltwort)** *Salsola kali L.* | *Salsola tragus L.*

*Akkadian: maštakal (šammu ša šamê šubatšu, "the plant whose home is heaven")*

Amaranthaceae | Whole plant, especially ash

**Taste:** Salty, bitter

**Temperature:** Cool

**Channels:** Kidney, Bladder, Skin (bath); Lung, Heart (fumigation)

**Planetary Ruler:** Moon, Saturn

**Element:** Water, Earth

The preeminent purification agent of Mesopotamian ritual pharmacology, *maštakal* represents archetypal Sky Medicine of the ancient Near East — a physical substance functioning as celestial emissary. The *Uruanna* lexicon identifies this alkali-rich halophyte as essential for dissolving spiritual pollution (*muššu*) from body and dwelling. When burned, the plant yields soapy alkaline ash capable of dissolving both physical impurity and the subtle residue of malevolent dream-spirits. The epithet "the plant whose home is heaven" indicates precise cosmological positioning: *maštakal* brings the purifying power of upper waters to the sublunary realm, serving as a conduit for Enki/Ea's cleansing force.

In oneiric application, the *āšipu* addressed conditions where dreams had deposited pathogenic residue upon the dreamer: nightmares leaving lingering pollution; prophetic dreams whose warning required ritual dissolution (*namburbi*); and invasive *zaqīqu* spirits attached to the client's subtle body. Decoctions prepared for ritual bathing at dawn, fumigation smoke for spatial cleansing, and preparations combining soapwort (*Saponaria officinalis*; Akkadian *kupatillû*), cedar (*Cedrus libani*; Akkadian *erēnu*), and tamarisk (*Tamarix* spp.; Akkadian *bīnu*) provided comprehensive liberation from oneiric contamination.

Symbolic formula proved as essential as biochemical action. Reciting "*šammu ša šamê šubatšu*" activated the plant's celestial power. Orientation toward the rising sun (Šamaš, judge of dreams) established cosmological positioning. Depending on ritual context, *maštakal* serves both apotropaic (omen-dissolving) and preparatory (dream-inviting) functions.

Modern correlates: glasswort (Salicornia europaea), soapwort (Saponaria officinalis), salt baths.
**Cautions.** Strongly alkaline ash requires careful dilution for external application. Internal use not indicated.

# General Opening and Intensification

**Mugwort** *Artemisia vulgaris L.*

Asteraceae | Aerial portions

**Taste:** Bitter, pungent

**Temperature:** Warm

**Channels:** Liver, Spleen, Kidney

**Planetary Ruler:** Moon

**Element:** Water

Preeminent oneirogen of the Northern Hemisphere. Named for Artemis, goddess of moon and wild places, lunar rulership positions mugwort as the foundational dream-opener — rendering the gates of sleep permeable. Thujone acts as a GABA receptor antagonist, producing mild cortical stimulation that maintains awareness during REM. Mugwort dreams feel more present: heightened awareness within the dream state rather than passive reception.

**Administration.** Olfactory (safest): dried herb in sachet beneath pillow. Internal: infusion (1 tsp per cup, steeped 10 minutes, taken 30 minutes before sleep) or tincture (15–30 drops). Topical: infused oil applied to temples.

**Cautions.** Pregnancy (emmenagogue). Lactation. Asteraceae allergy.

**Blue Lotus** *Nymphaea caerulea Savigny*

*Egyptian: sšn*

Nymphaeaceae | Flowers

**Taste:** Bitter, slightly sweet

**Temperature:** Cool

**Channels:** Heart, Liver, Kidney

**Planetary Ruler:** Venus

**Element:** Water

Sacred in Egyptian iconography — ubiquitous in temple art and funerary contexts. Venus rulership indicates function: receptive states where the dreamer opens to subtle communication rather than actively seeking. The flower's emergence from muddy waters to pristine bloom symbolizes spiritual transformation — the soul rising from material darkness into illuminated awareness. Contains apomorphine and nuciferine affecting dopamine receptors.

**Administration.** Traditional: 3–5g dried flowers steeped in wine for several hours. Aqueous infusion (15–20 minutes) provides milder effect.

**Cautions.** Legal status varies by jurisdiction. May potentiate sedatives. Avoid in pregnancy and lactation.

## Prophetic and Divinatory

**Dream Herb** *Calea zacatechichi Schltdl.*

*Chontal Maya: thle-pelakano ("leaf of god")*

Asteraceae | Leaves, aerial portions

**Taste:** Intensely bitter

**Temperature:** Warm

**Channels:** Liver, Heart

**Planetary Ruler:** Jupiter, Mercury

**Element:** Fire

Principal oneirogen of Mesoamerican tradition, employed by Chontal Maya for focused prophetic inquiry. The dual rulership of

Jupiter (expansion, prophecy) and Mercury (communication, specificity) indicates function: not merely to open gates but to direct prophetic faculty toward particular questions. No psychoactive alkaloids have been identified; mechanism unknown.

**Administration.** Infusion (1 tablespoon dried leaves, steeped 10–15 minutes) before sleep, sweetened with honey. Some practitioners smoke dried leaves. Formulate a specific question before consumption.

**Cautions.** Intense bitterness may cause nausea. Avoid in pregnancy and lactation.

**Bay Laurel** *Laurus nobilis L.*

Lauraceae | Leaves, essential oil

**Taste:** Pungent, bitter, aromatic

**Temperature:** Warm

**Channels:** Lung, Stomach, Spleen

**Planetary Ruler:** Sun

**Element:** Fire

Sacred to Apollo. The Pythia at Delphi reportedly chewed bay leaves before delivering oracles; the temple was wreathed in laurel. As a solar herb, bay provides clarity for interpreting symbolic content. Where mugwort opens gates, bay illuminates what is encountered. The two work synergistically: mugwort to induce vivid dreaming, bay to render symbolism intelligible.

**Administration.** One to three dried leaves beneath pillow before sleep, often with a specific question formulated. Combine with mugwort in dream sachets. Essential oil (diluted) applied to temples.

**Cautions.** Essential oil may cause skin sensitization. Large internal doses may irritate the gastrointestinal tract.

**Mandrake** *Mandragora officinarum L.*

*Akkadian: nam-tar ("fate-cutter")*

Solanaceae | Root, leaves, fruit (all toxic)

**Taste:** Bitter, acrid

**Temperature:** Cold

**Channels:** Heart, Liver

**Planetary Ruler:** Saturn (root), Venus (fruit)

**Element:** Earth

Central in Mesopotamian oneirobotany and prominent throughout medieval Europe, the Akkadian *nam-tar* ("fate-cutter") indicates ritual significance: the plant severs the thread binding the soul to waking consciousness. Contains tropane alkaloids (hyoscyamine, scopolamine) producing profound anticholinergic effects — sedation, amnesia, and at sufficient doses, vivid hallucination. Dioscorides describes sleep so deep that surgical operations could proceed without awareness.

Saturn's rulership positions mandrake among substances governing thresholds and communion with chthonic powers. Its coldness and capacity to induce profound unconsciousness make it inappropriate for general dream enhancement — it overwhelms natural sleep architecture. It belongs to a specialized incubation pharmacopoeia where complete dissociation from waking consciousness is the goal.

CAUTION: TOXIC. Medicine bag only; not for internal administration. All parts contain potentially lethal tropane alkaloids with a narrow margin between effective and toxic dose. Historical study only.

# Ancestral Communication

**African Dream Root** *Silene capensis Burm. f.*

*Xhosa: undlela ziimhlophe ("white paths")*

Caryophyllaceae | Root

**Taste:** Bland, slightly acrid

**Temperature:** Neutral

**Channels:** Heart, Kidney

**Planetary Ruler:** Saturn

**Element:** Earth

Principal oneirogen of the southern African *ubulawu* tradition. Saturn's rulership — planet of boundaries, thresholds, ancestors, and the dead — matches function precisely: illuminating paths between the living and the departed. The Xhosa name "white paths" describes the roads along which ancestors travel. No psychoactive compounds have been identified.

**Administration.** Traditional: half a teaspoon of powdered root vigorously stirred in cold water to produce white foam, consumed in the morning on an empty stomach. Effects manifest over the following nights. May be repeated for several days.

**Cautions.** Limited safety data. Begin with small doses. Traditional context emphasizes intention-setting and respect for ancestral protocols.

## Recall and Clarity

**Intellect Tree** *Celastrus paniculatus Willd.*

*Sanskrit: jyotiṣmatī* ज्योतिष्मती *("the luminous one")*

Celastraceae | Seeds, seed oil

**Rasa:** Tikta (bitter), Kaṭu (pungent)

**Vīrya:** Uṣṇa (hot)

**Planetary Ruler:** Mercury

**Element:** Fire

Chief among Āyurvedic *medhya rasāyana*. Mercury rulership indicates specific function: not to open gates or induce visions but to ensure the dreamer returns with the message intact. Where other oneirogens facilitate the journey, intellect tree illuminates the path home. The Sanskrit name derives from *jyotiṣ* (light) – the same root giving *jyotiṣa* (Vedic astrology). The plant illuminates mind as astrology illuminates fate.

**Administration.** Seeds: begin with one daily, increasing by one each day to a maximum of fifteen, then decrease. Seed oil: 5–15 drops in warm milk before sleep. Combines well with mugwort or African dream root to enhance recall.

**Cautions.** Large doses may cause gastrointestinal upset. Avoid in pregnancy. May aggravate Pitta.

**Polygala Root** *Polygala tenuifolia Willd.*

*Chinese: yuǎn zhì* 远志 *("far-reaching will")*

Polygalaceae | Root

**Taste:** Bitter, pungent

**Temperature:** Slightly warm

**Channels:** Heart, Kidney, Lung

**Planetary Ruler:** Mercury

**Element:** Water, Fire

Addresses the Heart-Kidney connection underlying both memory and prophetic capacity. Calms *shén*, opens Heart orifices blocked by phlegm, and facilitates Water-Fire communication essential for clear consciousness. Indicated where phlegm clouds dream clarity — patient dreams but cannot remember, or dreams feel murky and indistinct. Combines well with sour jujube seed.

**Administration.** Decoction: 3–9g.

**Cautions.** May irritate gastric mucosa. Contraindicated in gastric or duodenal ulcer.

## Substrate Restoration

**Sour Jujube Seed** *Ziziphus jujuba Mill. var. spinosa*

*Chinese: suān zǎo rén* 酸枣仁

Rhamnaceae | Seed

**Taste:** Sweet, sour

**Temperature:** Neutral

**Channels:** Heart, Liver, Gallbladder

**Planetary Ruler:** Jupiter

**Element:** Earth

Unlike oneirogens that directly induce dreams, sour jujube seed addresses the physiological substrate. Jupiter's rulership operates through the Liver/*hún* axis: nourishing Heart Blood provides a material basis for stable *shén* residence; calming Liver Yang allows *hún* to travel freely. Indicated where dream disturbance arises from deficiency — insomnia, excessive dreaming with fatigue, and inability to recall. Restore substrate before stimulating oneirogens can open gates.

**Administration.** Decoction: 9–18g. Powder: 3–6g before sleep. Raw form calms; dry-fried is more astringent.

**Cautions.** Excess heat. Severe damp-heat.

**Ashwagandha** *Withania somnifera (L.) Dunal*

Solanaceae | Root

**Rasa:** Tikta (bitter), Kaṣāya (astringent)

**Vīrya:** Uṣṇa (hot)

**Planetary Ruler:** Saturn, Mars

**Element:** Earth

The species name *somnifera* ("sleep-bearing") signals traditional use. As an adaptogen, ashwagandha normalizes stress response and supports adrenal function — addressing modern conditions underlying most sleep disturbance. Withanolides calm without sedating, enabling natural sleep architecture and REM periods where vivid dreaming occurs. Āyurveda classifies it as *rasāyana,* indicated for *vāta* disturbance — anxiety, restlessness, fragmented sleep. Grounding *vāta* creates stable conditions for coherent dreaming.

**Administration.** Root powder: 3–6g in warm milk before sleep. Tincture: 2–4ml. Best taken consistently over weeks for cumulative effect.

**Cautions.** May aggravate Pitta. Exercise caution in pregnancy. May potentiate sedatives and thyroid medications.

## Stabilization and Modulation

**Lavender** *Lavandula angustifolia Mill.*

Lamiaceae | Flowers, essential oil

**Taste:** Pungent, slightly bitter

**Temperature:** Cool

**Channels:** Heart, Liver, Lung

**Planetary Ruler:** Mercury

**Element:** Air

Primary oneiric function: purification and stabilization. Calming the nervous system and promoting sleep quality facilitates onset of REM sleep where complex and meaningful dreams occur. Acts as a moderating influence when combined with more stimulating oneirogens — maintaining the portal's accessibility while preventing disturbance. Mercury rulership speaks to mediatorial function: creating conditions for clear transmission of symbolic content. Particularly indicated where *hún* hyperactivity produces excessive, disturbing, or chaotic dreams.

**Administration.** Olfactory: sachets, pillow sprays, diffused essential oil. Infusion: 1 teaspoon dried flowers. Combines well with mugwort to moderate intensity.

**Cautions.** Essential oil may cause skin sensitization in some individuals.

*Table 14.1. Oneirogens: Taste, Temperature, Planetary Ruler, and Function*

| Plant | Taste | Temperature | Planet | Function |
|---|---|---|---|---|
| *Heavenly Plant (Prickly Saltwort)* | Salty, bitter | Cool | ☽ ♄ | Purification, apotropaic |
| *Mugwort* | Bitter, pungent | Warm | ☽ | General opening |
| *Blue Lotus* | Bitter, slightly sweet | Cool | ♀ | Receptive states |
| *Dream Herb* | Intensely bitter | Warm | ♃ ☿ | Prophetic, divinatory |
| *Bay Laurel* | Pungent, bitter | Warm | ☉ | Prophetic clarity |
| *Mandrake* | Bitter, acrid | Cold | ♄ ♀ | Threshold dissociation |
| *African Dream Root* | Bland, slightly acrid | Neutral | ♄ | Ancestral communion |
| *Intellect Tree* | Bitter, pungent | Hot | ☿ | Recall, clarity |
| *Polygala Root* | Bitter, pungent | Slightly warm | ☿ | Recall, phlegm-clearing |
| *Sour Jujube Seed* | Sweet, sour | Neutral | ♃ | Substrate restoration |
| *Ashwagandha* | Bitter, astringent | Hot | ♄ ♂ | Substrate, grounding |
| *Lavender* | Pungent, slightly bitter | Cool | ☿ | Stabilization, modulation |

# Celestial Selection

Planetary signatures guide clinical selection. Match the diagnostic picture to the plant whose celestial ruler addresses the condition.

When the diagnostic picture indicates need for general opening – the patient who does not dream, whose *hún* remains earthbound – mugwort under Moon provides foundational intervention. When specific questions require answers, dream herb under Jupiter and Mercury focuses prophetic faculty. When ancestral guidance is sought – inheritance disputes, family patterns requiring resolution – African dream root under Saturn illuminates paths between worlds.

Blue lotus under Venus serves where receptive states are indicated – the dreamer who needs to receive rather than seek. Sour jujube seed under Jupiter addresses the Liver/*hún* axis directly, rooting and clearing so better dreams arise from nourished substrate. Intellect tree under Mercury ensures the dreamer returns with the message intact.

Combine according to the diagnostic picture. The patient seeking ancestral guidance but struggling with recall: African dream root (Saturn) with intellect tree (Mercury). The depleted patient whose dreams have ceased: sour jujube seed to restore substrate before mugwort can open gates. Selection proceeds from principle rather than guesswork.

The correspondence between planet and function:

**Moon.** General opening. Rendering the threshold permeable. Mugwort.

**Mercury.** Recall and clarity. Ensuring the message returns intact. Intellect tree, polygala root, lavender.

**Venus.** Receptive states. Opening to subtle communication. Blue lotus.

**Sun.** Prophetic clarity. Illuminating symbolic content. Bay laurel.

**Jupiter.** Prophetic vision and substrate restoration. Dream herb, sour jujube seed.

**Saturn.** Ancestral communion and threshold work. African dream root, mandrake, ashwagandha.

## Biological Mechanisms

REM sleep runs on acetylcholine. Substances inhibiting acetylcholinesterase — the enzyme breaking down acetylcholine — intensify dream vividness and recall. Galantamine, derived from snowdrops (*Galanthus nivalis*), bridges traditional knowledge and contemporary pharmacology.

Thujone in mugwort acts as a GABA receptor antagonist, producing mild stimulation rather than sedation. In dreaming, this may maintain sufficient cortical activation for awareness while the body remains in REM atonia — the balance between sleep and waking that characterizes lucid dreaming. Traditional intuition that mugwort makes dreams "more real" correlates with this mechanism.

Scent bypasses cortical filtering, accessing the limbic system directly. Sleeping with aromatic herbs exploits this pathway. Tropane alkaloids in solanaceous plants act as muscarinic receptor antagonists. Blue lotus contains dopaminergic compounds. African dream root and dream herb remain pharmacologically unexplained — traditional knowledge identifying effects through pathways science has not yet characterized.

## The Plant Whose Home Is Heaven

The Mesopotamian formula returns us to first principles. *Šammu ša šamê šubatšu* — the plant whose home is heaven — names not merely a specific herb but the essential nature of all oneirogens. These substances belong to two worlds simultaneously. Rooted in earth, they carry celestial signatures. Administered to the body, they open gates of soul.

The practitioner who grasps this dual citizenship understands why selection cannot proceed by symptom-matching alone. The diagnostic picture must include the heavens.

Mesopotamian healers recognized what modern pharmacology obscures: dream disturbance arises from both physical imbalance and spiritual condition, requiring botanical and ritual response. The *āšipu* did not prescribe *maštakal* as we might prescribe a sedative. He positioned the dreamer within a cosmic framework — orientation toward Šamaš, invocation of Ea and Marduk, recitation of the plant's celestial name — so that the substance could function as bridge rather than mere biochemistry. Ritual context activated the plant's nature as emissary between realms.

This principle extends to all oneiric allies. Mugwort opens gates not because thujone modulates GABA receptors — though it does — but because Moon governs thresholds and *Artemisia* carries lunar signature into the body. African dream root illuminates ancestral paths not despite pharmacological opacity but because Saturn's influence operates through channels science has yet to map. The mechanisms matter. The correspondences matter more. Or rather: the correspondences are the deeper mechanism, of which biochemistry is the material expression.

The celestial medicine practitioner therefore selects plant allies as ancient practitioners did: reading the diagnostic picture through planetary lenses, matching the patient's condition to the substance whose ruling star addresses that condition, administering within a framework that honors the plant's dual nature. Moon for opening. Mercury for recall. Jupiter for prophecy. Saturn for ancestors. Venus for reception. Sun for illumination. The formula remains stable across four millennia because it describes real structure — the way consciousness, cosmos, and green allies actually interrelate.

In the silent hours when the *hún* takes flight and the *zaqīqu* travels between worlds, these allies stand ready. Each carries the light of its ruling star into the territory of sleep. Each opens, clarifies, or preserves according to its nature. The practitioner who knows their signatures can select precisely — not "a dream herb" but this dream herb, for this patient, at this moment in the unfolding pattern. The plant whose home is heaven meets the soul whose home is temporarily earth, and for a night, the distance between them closes.

## Sources


Abusch, Tzvi, and Karel van der Toorn, eds. Mesopotamian Magic. Groningen: Styx, 1999.

Bensky, Dan, Steven Clavey, and Erich Stöger. Chinese Herbal Medicine: Materia Medica. 3rd ed. Seattle: Eastland Press, 2004.

Butler, Sally A. L. Mesopotamian Conceptions of Dreams and Dream Rituals. Münster: Ugarit-Verlag, 1998.

Edelstein, Emma J., and Ludwig Edelstein. Asclepius. Baltimore: Johns Hopkins University Press, 1945.

Emboden, William A. "The Sacred Narcotic Lily of the Nile." Economic Botany 32 (1978): 395–407.

Frawley, David, and Vasant Lad. The Yoga of Herbs. Twin Lakes: Lotus Press, 2001.

Hirst, Manton. "Dreams and Medicines: Xhosa Diviners." Indo-Pacific Journal of Phenomenology 5 (2005): 1–22.

Mayagoitia, Lidia, et al. "Psychopharmacologic Analysis of Calea zacatechichi." Journal of Ethnopharmacology 18 (1986): 229–243.

Oppenheim, A. Leo. The Interpretation of Dreams in the Ancient Near East. Philadelphia: American Philosophical Society, 1956.

Scurlock, JoAnn, and Burton R. Andersen. Diagnoses in Assyrian and Babylonian Medicine. Urbana: University of Illinois Press, 2005.

Sharma, Priya Vrat, trans. Caraka Saṃhitā. Varanasi: Chaukhambha Orientalia, 1981–1994.

# Epilogue

*The dreamer dreams. The observer observes.*
*Through observation, awakening.*

The dreamer who dreams the dream awakens to the dream of all our lives within the central sun. The observer who observes awakens in the dream of this life. Through this awakening, we move toward spiritual liberation and self-realization. The frameworks assembled in these chapters serve this aim—not interpretation for its own sake, but recognition of who dreams and what dreaming serves.

This work has sought to excavate the use of astrology for understanding dreams—both as oracle and as signs along the way. The organ-spirits name what moves in the dreamer. The botanical allies open, clarify, preserve. The celestial signatures reveal pattern and meaning. Convergent streams, one practice.

For the practitioner, this increases capacity. Sky and dream share presence with the client. Unfurling memories, sorting experience, remembering futures. Distinguish the dream that diagnoses from the dream that prophesies from the dream that clears. Treat the root—and through treating, participate in another's awakening.

For the tradition, this means restoration. The Mesopotamian *āšipu* reading the *Iškar Zaqīqu*, the Greek *iatromantis* in the Asclepian *abaton*, the Daoist master practicing *Shuì Gōng*—each worked within integrated frameworks linking dream to cosmos to liberation. Modernity fragmented this unity. What was never separate can be rejoined. The lineages continue through those who practice.

Tonight, the sleeper will sleep. They will dream. Tomorrow they may speak of what arose—and in the speaking, the dreamer begins to observe; in the observing, the dreamer begins to awaken. The celestial medicine of dreams moves from page to practice, from practice to recognition, from recognition toward the central sun.

# APPENDICES

## Part I: Reference Tables

### Appendix A

# Dream Symbol Concordance

# Using This Concordance

Part One offers planetary and elemental attributions for common dream symbols, drawn from Artemidorus, Bonatti, Agrippa, Vedic tradition, and clinical observation. Part Two presents cross-cultural comparisons across Classical Mediterranean, Islamic (Ibn Sirin), Chinese (Zhou Gong), and Indigenous traditions.

Identify significant symbols from the dream and locate them in Part One for planetary attribution, then consult Part Two for cross-cultural resonance. Where traditions converge, interpretation gains confidence. Where they diverge, the dreamer's cultural background and personal associations determine which lens applies. The dream chart provides celestial context that transcends cultural boundaries.

Abbreviations: Sun, Moon, Mercury, Venus, Mars, Jupiter, Saturn. Elements: F (Fire), E (Earth), A (Air), W (Water).

# Interpretive Principles

## *Dual-Element Symbols*

Some symbols bridge two elements, indicated by notation like F/W (Fire/Water). Banquet (F/W) combines Fire's expansive celebration with Water's emotional communion. Blood (W/F) flows like water but carries fire's vital heat. Cave (E/W) holds earth's structure while containing water's hidden depths. Interpretation should consider which element dominates in the specific dream context.

## *Multi-Rulership Symbols*

Symbols with multiple planetary rulers (e.g., Bear Mars/Saturn, Serpent Moon/Saturn/Mercury) bring all influences into play. The Bear combines Mars's strength and aggression with Saturn's solitude and hibernation. The Serpent unites Moon's unconscious depths, Saturn's chthonic wisdom, and Mercury's transformative cunning.

# Part One: Alphabetical Concordance

The following concordance organizes dream symbols by their planetary and elemental attributions.

*Table A.1. Dream Concordance*

| Symbol | Planet | Elem | Traditional Meaning |
|---|---|---|---|
| **Altar** | ♃/☉ | F | Sacred matters, religious calling, sacrifice required |
| **Ancestors** | ♄ | E | Karmic themes, inheritance, family patterns |
| **Armor** | ♂ | F | Protection needed, defensiveness, preparation for conflict |
| **Ashes** | ♄ | E | Endings, purification complete, transformation residue |
| **Baby** | ☽ | W | New beginnings, vulnerability, potential, the nascent |
| **Banquet** | ♃ | F/W | Abundance, celebration, social success, excess |
| **Bath** | ♀/☽ | W | Purification, sensuality, emotional cleansing |
| **Bear** | ♂/♄ | E | Strength, maternal protection, hibernation, solitude |
| **Bed** | ♀/☽ | W | Rest, intimacy, illness, the marriage state |
| **Birds** | ☿ | A | Messages, thoughts, spirit, freedom, news coming |
| **Blood** | ♂ | W/F | Life force, injury, kinship, sacrifice, passion |
| **Boat/Ship** | ☽ | W | Life journey, emotional passage, the body |
| **Book** | ☿/♃ | A | Knowledge, record, memory, contracts, learning |
| **Bridge** | ☿ | A | Transition, connection, crossing between states |
| **Bull** | ♀ | E | Fertility, stubbornness, material wealth, Taurus |
| **Burial** | ♄ | E | Endings, the unconscious, secrets, transformation |
| **Candle** | ☉/♂ | F | Consciousness, prayer, life span, illumination |
| **Castle** | ♄/☉ | E/F | Ambition, protection, authority, the self |
| **Cat** | ☽/♀ | W | Independence, intuition, feminine mystery, sensuality |
| **Cave** | ♄/☽ | E/W | The unconscious, womb, retreat, hidden knowledge |
| **Child** | ☽/☉ | W/F | Innocence, potential, the inner child, new projects |
| **Church** | ♃ | F | Spiritual life, community, tradition, sanctuary |
| **Clock** | ♄ | E | Time pressure, mortality, timing, patience required |
| **Clothing** | ♀/☽ | A/W | Persona, social role, covering, how one appears |
| **Clouds** | ☽/♃ | A/W | Obscured truth, transition, fertility (rain-bringing) |
| **Corpse** | ♄ | E | Transformation, ending, the shadow, defunct situation |

| | | | |
|---|---|---|---|
| **Cow** | ☽/♀ | E/W | Nourishment, mother, prosperity, patience |
| **Crossroads** | ☿/♄ | E/A | Decision point, Hecate, choice, fate intersection |
| **Crown** | ☉ | F | Authority, achievement, the Self, highest aspiration |
| **Darkness** | ♄/☽ | W | The unknown, depression, the unconscious, gestation |
| **Death figure** | ♄ | E | Transformation, ending, initiation, the threshold |
| **Desert** | ♂/♄ | F/E | Spiritual trial, isolation, purification, barrenness |
| **Dog** | ♂/☽ | F/W | Loyalty, instinct, guardian, guide to underworld |
| **Door** | ☽/☿ | A | Opportunity, transition, threshold, access |
| **Dove** | ♀ | A | Peace, love, spirit, message, gentle communication |
| **Dragon** | ♂/♄ | F | Primal power, guardian, transformation, treasure |
| **Eagle** | ☉/♃ | F/A | Vision, spirit, authority, far-seeing, ambition |
| **Earthquake** | ♄/♂ | E | Foundation shaking, upheaval, structural change |
| **Egg** | ☽ | W | Potential, wholeness, fertility, the cosmic egg |
| **Eye** | ☉ | F | Consciousness, perception, the divine watching, truth |
| **Father** | ☉/♄ | F/E | Authority, tradition, protection, discipline, origin |
| **Feast** | ♃/♀ | F/W | Abundance, celebration, integration, communion |
| **Fire** | ♂/☉ | F | Transformation, passion, anger, purification, spirit |
| **Fish** | ☽/♃ | W | The unconscious, Christianity, fertility, abundance |
| **Flood** | ☽/♄ | W | Overwhelm, purification, emotion, collective unconscious |
| **Flower** | ♀ | A/W | Beauty, transience, offering, growth, sexuality |
| **Forest/Woods** | ♄/☽ | E/W | The unconscious, nature, getting lost, primal self |
| **Fountain** | ♀/☽ | W | Life source, emotion, creativity, the feminine |
| **Fox** | ☿ | F/A | Cunning, trickery, adaptability, cleverness |
| **Fruit** | ♀/♃ | E/W | Results, reward, fertility, sensual pleasure |
| **Garden** | ♀ | E/W | Cultivation, paradise, the soul, inner work results |
| **Gate** | ♄/☿ | E/A | Threshold, opportunity, guardian, access point |
| **Giant** | ♃/♄ | F/E | Overwhelming force, inflation, archetypal power |
| **Gold** | ☉ | F | The Self, highest value, solar consciousness, wealth |
| **Grave** | ♄ | E | Endings, the past, ancestors, transformation, rest |
| **Hair** | ♀/☽ | A/W | Vitality, sexuality, thoughts, social identity |
| **Hand** | ☿ | A | Agency, skill, giving/receiving, blessing, work |
| **Heart** | ☉/♀ | F/W | Center, love, courage, truth, the essential self |
| **Horse** | ♂/♃ | F | Instinct, power, freedom, nobility, the body |
| **Hospital** | ☽/♃ | W | Healing need, vulnerability, care, transition |
| **House** | ☽/♄ | E/W | The self, the body, family, security, psyche structure |
| **Ice** | ♄ | W/E | Frozen emotion, stasis, preservation, coldness |
| **Island** | ☽/♄ | E/W | Isolation, refuge, the self, individuation |

| | | | |
|---|---|---|---|
| **Jewels** | ☉/♀ | F/E | Value, the Self, spiritual attainment, treasure |
| **Journey** | ☿/☽ | A | Life path, process, quest, transformation underway |
| **Judge** | ♃/♄ | A/E | Conscience, authority, evaluation, karma |
| **Key** | ☿/♄ | A/E | Access, solution, knowledge, power over entry |
| **King** | ☉ | F | The Self, authority, solar consciousness, mastery |
| **Knife** | ♂ | F | Discrimination, severance, aggression, surgery |
| **Ladder** | ☿/♃ | A | Ascent, progress, hierarchy, connection above/below |
| **Lake** | ☽ | W | The unconscious, reflection, contained emotion, depth |
| **Letter** | ☿ | A | Message, news, communication, contract, fate |
| **Light** | ☉ | F | Consciousness, revelation, divine presence, clarity |
| **Lightning** | ♂/♃ | F/A | Sudden insight, divine intervention, destruction/illumination |
| **Lion** | ☉ | F | Nobility, courage, solar power, the heart, Leo |
| **Lock** | ♄ | E | Obstruction, secret, protection, closure |
| **Marriage/Wedding** | ♀/♃ | W/F | Union, commitment, integration of opposites, celebration |
| **Mask** | ☽/☿ | A | Persona, deception, hidden identity, role |
| **Medicine** | ☿/♃ | A/W | Healing, remedy, transformation agent, the cure |
| **Mirror** | ☽/♀ | W/A | Self-reflection, truth, vanity, the soul image |
| **Money** | ♀/♃ | E | Value, energy, exchange, worth, resources |
| **Monster** | ♂/♄ | F/E | Shadow, fear, repressed content, threshold guardian |
| **Moon** | ☽ | W | The feminine, cycles, the unconscious, mother |
| **Mother** | ☽ | W | The feminine, origin, nurture, nature, the unconscious |
| **Mountain** | ♄/♃ | E/A | Aspiration, achievement, obstacle, the Self, overview |
| **Mud** | ♄/☽ | E/W | Confusion, prima materia, potential, stuck situation |
| **Nakedness** | ☽/♀ | W | Vulnerability, truth, exposure, naturalness, shame |
| **Night** | ☽/♄ | W | The unconscious, hidden things, gestation, rest |
| **Ocean/Sea** | ☽/♃ | W | The collective unconscious, mother, infinity, origin |
| **Old man** | ♄ | E | Wisdom, the Senex, time, limitation, death |
| **Old woman** | ♄/☽ | E/W | Wisdom, the Crone, fate, the unconscious, death |
| **Path/Road** | ☿ | A/E | Life direction, the Way, choice, journey, process |
| **Pearl** | ☽ | W | Wisdom from suffering, the feminine, lunar treasure |
| **Physician** | ☿/♃ | A | The healer, Mercury, remedy, diagnosis, guidance |
| **Pig** | ♀/☽ | E/W | Fertility, greed, earthiness, abundance, instinct |
| **Poison** | ♄/♂ | W | Danger, transformation, hidden threat, medicine (dose) |
| **Pregnancy** | ☽ | W | Creativity, potential, development, new life forming |
| **Priest** | ♃ | F/A | Spirit, authority, mediation, blessing, teaching |
| **Prison** | ♄ | E | Restriction, karma, depression, shadow work needed |

| | | | |
|---|---|---|---|
| **Queen** | ☽/♀ | W | The feminine Self, receptivity, soul, inner authority |
| **Rain** | ☽/♃ | W/A | Blessing, fertility, emotion, grace, cleansing |
| **Rainbow** | ☉/☽ | A/W | Promise, bridge, wholeness, divine covenant |
| **Rat** | ♄/☿ | E | Survival, disease, the shadow, gnawing anxiety |
| **Raven/Crow** | ♄ | A | Death, transformation, prophecy, the shadow |
| **Ring** | ♀/♄ | E | Commitment, wholeness, eternity, bond, the Self |
| **River** | ☽ | W | Life flow, time, emotion, boundary, transition |
| **Rock/Stone** | ♄ | E | Permanence, obstacle, foundation, the Self (lapis) |
| **Rose** | ♀ | W/F | Love, beauty, the feminine, heart, secrecy (sub rosa) |
| **Sacrifice** | ♂/♄ | F | Transformation, letting go, offering, exchange |
| **School** | ☿/♃ | A | Learning, testing, development, life lessons |
| **Seed** | ♄/☽ | E | Potential, beginning, essence, karma, inheritance |
| **Serpent/Snake** | ☽/♄/☿ | E/W | Transformation, wisdom, danger, kundalini, healing |
| **Shadow (figure)** | ♄ | E | The rejected self, unconscious, what follows |
| **Silver** | ☽ | W | The feminine, reflection, lunar consciousness, value |
| **Skeleton** | ♄ | E | Death, structure, the essential, mortality |
| **Sky** | ♃/☉ | A/F | Spirit, the divine, aspiration, overview, heaven |
| **Spider** | ♄/☽ | A/E | Fate weaving, patience, the feminine, creation/trap |
| **Stairs** | ☿/♃ | A | Progress, ascent/descent, levels, transition |
| **Star** | ☉/♃ | F/A | Destiny, hope, guidance, the divine spark |
| **Storm** | ♂/♃ | A/W | Upheaval, emotion, cleansing, divine power |
| **Stranger** | ☿/♄ | A | Unknown aspect of self, new potential, threat |
| **Sun** | ☉ | F | Consciousness, the Self, vitality, the divine, father |
| **Sword** | ♂ | F/A | Discrimination, conflict, truth, power, decision |
| **Teacher** | ♃/☿ | A/F | Guidance, wisdom, authority, the inner teacher |
| **Teeth (losing)** | ♄ | E | Loss, aging, powerlessness, foundation problems |
| **Temple** | ♃/☉ | F | Sacred center, the Self, spiritual aspiration |
| **Thief** | ☿/♂ | A | Loss, shadow, trickster, taking what isn't yours |
| **Throne** | ☉/♃ | F | Authority, the Self, achievement, power |
| **Tiger** | ♂ | F | Power, passion, danger, instinct, aggression |
| **Tomb** | ♄ | E | Death, transformation, the womb/tomb, initiation |
| **Tower** | ♄/♂ | E/F | Ambition, isolation, structure, destruction (falling) |
| **Train** | ♄/☿ | E/A | Collective journey, fate track, scheduled path |
| **Treasure** | ☉/♃ | E/F | The Self, hidden value, spiritual attainment |
| **Tree** | ♄/♃ | E | Life, growth, the Self, genealogy, world axis |
| **Underground** | ♄/☽ | E/W | The unconscious, death, hidden treasures, roots |
| **Unicorn** | ☽/♀ | A/W | Purity, the untamable, lunar femininity, magic |
| **Valley** | ☽/♀ | E/W | Receptivity, the feminine, shadow, depression |

| | | | |
|---|---|---|---|
| **Volcano** | ♂ | F/E | Eruption, suppressed anger, transformation, power |
| **Wall** | ♄ | E | Boundary, defense, obstacle, limitation |
| **War** | ♂ | F | Conflict, inner struggle, aggression, competition |
| **Water (clear)** | ☽ | W | Emotion, the unconscious, purity, life |
| **Water (muddy)** | ☽/♄ | W/E | Confused emotion, unconscious unclear, trouble |
| **Well** | ☽/♄ | W/E | Deep unconscious, source, feminine depths, wishing |
| **Whale** | ☽/♃ | W | The unconscious, containment, rebirth (Jonah), depth |
| **Wheel** | ♃/♄ | F/E | Fate, cycles, fortune, karma, wholeness |
| **Wind** | ☿ | A | Spirit, change, communication, the invisible |
| **Wine** | ♀/♃ | W | Spirit, celebration, transformation, intoxication |
| **Wings** | ☿ | A | Transcendence, spirit, freedom, aspiration |
| **Witch** | ☽/♄ | W/E | Feminine power, shadow, magic, transformation |
| **Wolf** | ♂/♄ | F/E | Instinct, the predator, pack, guardian, devourer |
| **Womb** | ☽ | W | Origin, potential, gestation, the feminine, return |
| **Wound** | ♂/♄ | F/W | Injury, vulnerability, the wounded healer, karma |
| **Youth** | ☿/♀ | A | Potential, the puer, energy, innocence, new |

# Part Two: Cross-Cultural Symbol Analysis

The following tables examine six universal dream symbols across four interpretive traditions: Classical, Islamic, Chinese, and Indigenous.

## *The Serpent*

*Table A.2. The Serpent across traditions.*

| Tradition | Interpretation |
|---|---|
| Classical | Chthonic wisdom; healing; danger; treasure guardian |
| Islamic | Enemy or deceiver; wealth if possessed; cure if killed |
| Chinese | Dragon transformation; wealth; pregnancy; ancestors |
| Indigenous | Rainbow Serpent-creator, water, fertility; vision ally |

## Water

*Table A.3. Water across traditions.*

| Tradition | Interpretation |
|---|---|
| Classical | Primordial chaos; clear = fortune; murky = trouble |
| Islamic | Blessing; pure religion; rain = divine mercy |
| Chinese | Clear = wealth; murky = lawsuit; flooding = Kidney yang deficiency |
| Indigenous | Sacred dwelling of spirits; Dreamtime waterhole |

## Teeth (Loss)

*Table A.4. Teeth (Loss) across traditions.*

| Tradition | Interpretation |
|---|---|
| Classical | Death of family member; loss of property |
| Islamic | Relatives; falling = death or separation |
| Chinese | Relatives' death; Kidney essence depletion |
| Indigenous | Loss of power; initiation; ancestors calling |

## Fire

*Table A.5. Fire across traditions.*

| Tradition | Interpretation |
|---|---|
| Classical | Transformation; passion; purification |
| Islamic | Trial; divine wrath; light = knowledge |
| Chinese | Heart fire; success/destruction; fever prodrome |
| Indigenous | Spirit contact; ceremonial power; cleansing |

## Flight

*Table A.6. Flight across traditions.*

| Tradition | Interpretation |
|---|---|
| Classical | Freedom; ambition; if too high = hubris |
| Islamic | Elevation in status; spiritual ascent |
| Chinese | Great success; hun-soul traveling; Liver qi rising |
| Indigenous | Shamanic journey; soul flight; acquiring allies |

## Mountain

*Table A.7. Mountain across traditions.*

| Tradition | Interpretation |
|---|---|
| Classical | Obstacle; achievement; celestial bridge |
| Islamic | Soul's challenges; summit = goal attained |
| Chinese | Career triumph; ancestors' graves; stability |
| Indigenous | Spirit dwelling; vision quest site; axis mundi |

## Summary

*Table A.8. Six symbols across four traditions.*

| Symbol | Classical | Islamic | Chinese | Indigenous |
|---|---|---|---|---|
| Serpent | Wisdom, healing | Enemy, betrayal | Dragon transform | Creator being |
| Water | Primordial chaos | Blessing | Wealth (clear) | Sacred dwelling |
| Teeth | Family death | Lineage loss | Relatives' death | Power loss |
| Fire | Transformation | Purification | Success/ destruction | Spirit contact |
| Flight | Freedom, ambition | Spiritual elevation | Great success | Shamanic journey |
| Mountain | Celestial bridge | Soul challenges | Career triumph | Spirit dwelling |

## Part Three: Elemental Symbol Categories

The classical elements organize vast categories of dream imagery according to their essential qualities.

### *Fire Symbols*

Flames, burning, sunlight, lightning, candles, torches, hearths, forges, volcanoes, fever, anger, passion, illumination, gold, red and orange colors, lions, salamanders, dragons, phoenixes, the heart, noon, summer, transformation, purification.

### *Water Symbols*

Oceans, rivers, lakes, rain, tears, blood, wine, milk, baths, wells, floods, drowning, ships, fish, dolphins, whales, silver, blue and green colors, the womb, emotions, dreams within dreams, dissolution, the unconscious.

### *Air Symbols*

Wind, breath, clouds, storms, flying, birds, butterflies, feathers, smoke, incense, high places, towers, lungs, voice, yellow colors, dawn, spring, communication, thought, messages, the mental realm.

### *Earth Symbols*

Soil, stones, mountains, caves, fields, gardens, trees, roots, bones, buildings, walls, foundations, graves, seeds, harvests, cattle, brown and black colors, midnight, winter, the body, stability, manifestation.

## Part Four: Reverse Index by Planet

When a planet dominates the dream chart by rulership, aspect, or angularity, consult its symbol list for interpretive resonance.

## Sun

Authority figures, kings, fathers, gold, lions, eagles, sunlight, crowns, thrones, palaces, hearts, eyes, the right side, circles, daylight hours, temples, laurel, heliotrope, chrysolite, frankincense, high places, centers, noon.

## Moon

Mothers, queens, women generally, silver, water, tides, mirrors, pearls, shells, crabs, owls, cats, the left side, breasts, stomach, ovaries, menstruation, pregnancy, infants, night travel, ships, fishermen, innkeepers, nurses, the public, crowds, wandering, changeability, crescents, Monday, white flowers, selenite, camphor, willow, cucumber, mushrooms.

## Mercury

Messengers, scribes, merchants, physicians, thieves, tricksters, youths, siblings, books, letters, documents, contracts, numbers, calculations, roads, crossroads, marketplaces, schools, hands, tongue, lungs, nervous system, birds, snakes, twins, mixed colors, Wednesday, lavender, marjoram, agate, quicksilver, communication devices, puzzles, codes.

## Venus

Lovers, young women, wives, artists, musicians, beautiful persons, copper, jewelry, flowers, gardens, orchards, bedchambers, baths, perfume, doves, swans, sparrows, rabbits, the throat, kidneys, veins, embraces, kisses, dancing, silk, green and soft colors, Friday, roses, myrtle, apple, emerald, turquoise, sugar, honey, pleasure houses, weddings.

## Mars

Soldiers, warriors, surgeons, butchers, smiths, enemies, competitors, brothers, iron, weapons, knives, fire, blood, wounds, battles, arguments, red colors, Tuesday, wolves, rams, scorpions, the head, muscles, adrenal glands, genitals (male), fevers, inflammation, forges, barracks, slaughterhouses, garlic, pepper, nettles, iron filings, ruby, bloodstone, thistle.

## *Jupiter*

Judges, priests, teachers, wealthy persons, benefactors, fathers (as provider), tin, large animals, horses, elephants, whales, eagles (as king of birds), the liver, thighs, growth, expansion, blue and purple, Thursday, oak, fig, nutmeg, sapphire, amethyst, cedar, churches, universities, courts of law, banquets, ceremonies, foreign lands, philosophy, religion, wealth.

## *Saturn*

Elders, grandparents, ancestors, the dead, hermits, farmers, miners, beggars, cripples, lead, stones, bones, earth, graves, ruins, prisons, monasteries, caves, mines, the skeleton, knees, spleen, teeth, skin, chronic conditions, black and dark colors, Saturday, cypress, yew, hemlock, onyx, obsidian, coal, ash, old buildings, clocks, hourglasses, boundaries, limits, endings, karma.

## *North Node (Rahu)*

In Vedic tradition, Rahu (the Dragon's Head) represents desire, ambition, worldly attachment, and the unfamiliar. Dreams featuring: foreign lands, exotic figures, outsiders, technological novelty, amplification and exaggeration, obsessive pursuit, masks and disguises, smoke and fog, eclipses, illusions that seduce, appetite without satisfaction, the new and untried, boundary violations, taboo-breaking, sudden elevation. Rahu dreams often indicate karmic areas requiring development in this lifetime-unfamiliar territory the soul must explore.

## *South Node (Ketu)*

In Vedic tradition, Ketu (the Dragon's Tail) represents liberation, detachment, past-life patterns, and spiritual insight. Dreams featuring: ancestors, past-life imagery, deja vu, familiar strangers, spiritual teachers, renunciation, loss that liberates, endings that free, flags and banners, headless figures, dissolution of boundaries, psychic phenomena, mystical experiences, things falling away. Ketu dreams often indicate karmic patterns carried from previous experience-gifts and burdens already developed.

# Appendix B

# Egyptian Astronomical Framework

# The Sidereal Architecture of the Night

Egyptian oneiromancy operated within a precise astronomical framework. The timing of a dream—which hour of the night, under which decan, during which phase of Ra's underworld journey—determined its significance and shaped its interpretation. This appendix presents the technical components of that framework for reference and application.

## I. The Two Classes of Stars

Egyptian astronomy divided the night sky into two primary groups, each with distinct oneiromantic significance.

### *Ikhemu-sek:* The Imperishable Stars

The northern circumpolar stars—those that never set below the horizon—were called *ikhemu-sek*, the 'Imperishables' or 'Indestructibles.' These stars served as the template for immortality. The pyramid shafts were aligned to them so the pharaoh's *ka* could join their eternal circuit.

Around 2500 BCE, Egyptian astronomers used the alignment of Kochab (Beta Ursae Minoris) and Mizar (Zeta Ursae Majoris) to determine True North with remarkable precision—essential for the astronomical orientation of temples and tombs.

*Constitutional correspondence:* The Horian type aligns with the Imperishable Stars. Dreams occurring when circumpolar stars dominate—during winter nights when they wheel highest—carry themes of permanence, divine kingship, and eternal order.

### *Ikhemu-wredj:* The Unwearying Stars

The southern stars that rise in the east and set in the west were called *ikhemu-wredj*, the 'Unwearying Ones.' These stars were perceived as passengers on the night boat of Ra during his twelve-hour voyage through the underworld.

This group includes the belt of thirty-six decans used for chronometry and the major constellations of *Sah* (Orion) and *Sopdet* (Sirius). The heliacal rising of *Sopdet*—when Sirius first becomes visible before dawn after a period of invisibility—signaled the annual flooding of the Nile and the start of the new year.

*Constitutional correspondence:* The Sethian type aligns with *Meskhetyu* (the Big Dipper), depicted in Egyptian star maps as the Foreleg of the Bull, often shown bound by chains and guarded by a hippopotamus goddess. Even the stars must be restrained from Seth's chaos.

Dreams occurring when southern stars dominate carry themes of transit, change, cyclical renewal, and the journey through darkness toward rebirth.

## II. The Thirty-Six Decans

The decans (from Greek *dekanos*, 'chief of ten') are star groups that rise consecutively to mark the progression of time throughout the night. The rising of each decan marked the beginning of a new 'hour,' creating a sidereal clock in use by at least the Tenth Dynasty (c. 2100 BCE).

The Egyptian year was a 'Living Star Calendar' of thirty-six weeks of ten days each, plus five epagomenal days for the birthdays of the gods. The entire system was anchored by the heliacal rising of *Sopdet*.

For oneiromantic purposes, the decan rising at the time of the dream—or the decan ruling the hour—influences the dream's quality and meaning.

*Table B.1. The thirty-six decans and oneiromantic values.*

| # | Transliteration | Translation | Oneiromantic Value |
|---|---|---|---|
| 1 | Tepy-a Kenmet | Predecessor of the Cow | New beginnings; jubilation; inception |
| 2 | Kenmet | The Cow | Development; growth; nurturing |
| 3 | Khery Heped Kenmet | Under the Hindquarters of the Cow | Change in circumstances; transformation |
| 4 | Hat Djat | Beginning of the Crane | Construction; building; foundations |
| 5 | Pehuy Djat | End of the Crane | Accomplishment; completion of work |
| 6 | Temat Heret | Upper Wing | Care; protection; sheltering |
| 7 | Temat Kheret | Lower Wing | Death; endings; completion |
| 8 | Weshati Bekati | The Pregnant Twins | Fertility; sexuality; duality |
| 9 | Ip-Djes | Recovered Senses | Service; restoration of clarity |
| 10 | Tepy-a Khentet | Predecessor of Khentet | Truth; justice; preparation |
| 11 | Khentet Heret | Upper Khentet | Chaos; disorder; disruption |
| 12 | Khentet Kheret | Lower Khentet | Conflict; war; struggle |
| 13 | Tjemes en Khentet | Red One of Khentet | Restraint; end of conflict; truce |
| 14 | Qedty | Band of Reeds | Sowing seeds; planting intentions |
| 15 | Hery-ib Wia | Middle of the Boat | Journey through life; passage |
| 16 | Seshmu | Guides; Winepress | Spiritual struggles; transformation |
| 17 | Kenmu | Secret Stars | Rest; repose; hidden matters |
| 18 | Tepy-a Semed | Predecessor of the Horn | Wisdom; tree of life; preparation |
| 19 | Semed | The Horn | Celebration; merriment; abundance |
| 20 | Seret | The Sheep | Melancholy; sadness; introspection |

| # | Transliteration | Translation | Oneiromantic Value |
|---|---|---|---|
| 21 | Sawy Seret | Children of the Sheep | Healing; restoration; recovery |
| 22 | Khery Heped Seret | Under the Hindquarters of the Sheep | Love; romance; relationships |
| 23 | Tepy-a Akhuy | Predecessor of the Two Spirits | Mixed blessings; ambivalence |
| 24 | Akhuy | The Two Spirits | Harvesting rewards; reaping |
| 25 | Bawy | The Two Souls | Abundance; spiritual wealth |
| 26 | Khentu Heru | Upper Khentu | Destruction of enemies; victory |
| 27 | Khentu Kheru | Lower Khentu | Authority; power; dominion |
| 28 | Qed | The Potter | Creation; artistry; shaping |
| 29 | Sawy Qed | Children of the Potter | Possessiveness; sharing; inheritance |
| 30 | Khau | Thousands | Respect; admiration; multitudes |
| 31 | Aryt | Roll of Papyrus | Writing; legacy; records |
| 32 | Remen Hery Sah | Upper Arm of Sah | Purification; cleansing; preparation |
| 33 | Remen Khery Sah | Lower Arm of Sah | Illumination; revelation; insight |
| 34 | Sah | The Father of Gods (Orion) | Protection; divine authority |
| 35 | Tepy-a Sopdet | Predecessor of Sopdet | Destruction of chaos; ordering |
| 36 | Sopdet | Goddess of the Flood (Sirius) | Inundation; abundance; renewal |

A dream occurring under the governance of *Sawy Seret* (decan 21) carries primary themes of healing and neutralization of disease. A dream during a *Khentet* hour signals chaotic influences requiring protective response. This method represents the earliest form of sidereal astrology, where 'hour markers' focused on the rising decan rather than the twelve zodiacal signs introduced later in the Ptolemaic period.

# III. The Twelve Hours of the Underworld

The twelve hours of the night were not merely chronological markers but mythological stages in the journey of the sun god Ra through the *Duat* (underworld). The 'Books of the Afterlife'—the *Amduat, Book of Gates,* and related texts—describe the trials and transformations occurring in each hour, providing a template for the dreamer's own visionary journey.

*Table B.2. The twelve hours and their qualities.*

| Hour | Mythological Event | Oneiromantic Quality |
|---|---|---|
| 1 | Ra enters the western horizon | Threshold crossing; beginning descent |
| 2 | Passage through Wernes | Fertile fields; abundance imagery |
| 3 | Waters of Osiris | 'Who cuts up souls'; nightmare territory |
| 4 | Desert of Rosetau | Barren passage; testing; endurance |
| 5 | Isis ignites the cavern fires | Transformative fire; purification |
| 6 | Ra and Osiris unite in the Nun | Deepest mystery; revelatory epiphany |
| 7 | Isis and the Elder Magician protect the flame | Defense against Apep; protective dreams |
| 8 | Clothing the forms | Identity; appearance; social role |
| 9 | Rowing toward the east | Effort; progress; approaching dawn |
| 10 | Drowning of enemies | Victory over opposition; resolution |
| 11 | Preparation for rebirth | Anticipation; readiness; gathering strength |
| 12 | Ra emerges as Khepri | Rebirth; renewal; dawn consciousness |

## *The Sixth Hour Mystery*

The deepest part of the night—the sixth hour—constitutes the most potent oneiromantic window. In this hour, Ra's *ba* (soul) and body, which separated at sunset, rejoin as the Death God Osiris. This unified deity is immersed in the *Nun* (primordial waters), tapping into the eternal energy of the beginning to facilitate rebirth at dawn.

Dreams occurring during the sixth hour were treated as revelatory epiphanies of the highest order, offering solutions to profound ailments or insights into cosmic truth. The sixth hour corresponds roughly to midnight—the pivot point of the night.

### *The Third Hour Warning*

The third hour—called 'Who cuts up souls'—represents nightmare territory. Dreams in this period were scrutinized for demonic influence and often required protective response rather than standard interpretation. Nightmares occurring here were differentiated from the purifying visions of the fifth hour or the defensive dreams of the seventh.

## IV. Planetary Personifications

The five visible planets (*akhemu-wredj*, 'stars that never rest') were personified as specific deities whose mythological traits modified the prognostic value of oneiromantic visions.

*Table B.3. Planetary personifications.*

| Planet | Egyptian Name | Iconography | Oneiromantic Realm |
|---|---|---|---|
| Jupiter | Horus Who Limits the Two Lands | Falcon-headed | Expansion; sanctifying sovereignty |
| Saturn | Horus the Bull of Heaven | Ox-headed | Stability; crossing the vault |
| Mars | Horus the Red | Triple snake-headed falcon | Blood; retrograde ('going backward') |
| Mercury | Sebegu (Seth) | Falcon with Seth-head | Twilight transition; unpredictability |
| Venus | The Phoenix / Osiris | Two-headed human or heron | Morning herald; horizon-crossing |

### *Mercury and Seth*

The identification of Mercury with Seth carries particular significance for dream interpretation. Dreams occurring during strong Mercurial influence—when Mercury is visible, angular, or ruling the hour—were scrutinized for Typhonian qualities: sudden disruptions, 'thunderstorm' temperaments, flaring of internal heat, deception, and boundary violations.

For Sethian constitutional types, Mercury's influence may prove favorable—native chaos meeting celestial chaos in productive resonance. For Horian types, the same influence signals disruption requiring protective measures.

### *The Horian Planets*

Jupiter, Saturn, and Mars all bear Horus epithets, ensuring their influences—though potentially harsh (as with 'Horus the Red')—remain within the protective framework of legitimate kingship and *Maat*. Dreams under these planets address themes of authority, stability, and right action, even when the imagery involves conflict or challenge.

## V. Application to Dream Interpretation

To apply this framework:

1. *Determine the hour.* Identify which of the twelve hours contains the dream time. Note the mythological stage of Ra's journey and the corresponding oneiromantic quality.
2. *Identify the ruling decan.* If possible, determine which decan was rising or ruling the hour. Cross-reference with Table B.1 for thematic influence.
3. *Note planetary visibility.* Which planets were visible? Was Mercury (Seth) prominent? This affects both constitutional interpretation and the dream's character.
4. *Apply constitutional filter.* The same astronomical configuration means differently for Horian and Sethian types. A sixth-hour dream under Mercury for a Sethian may bring revelation; for a

Horian, the same configuration may bring confusion requiring protective response.

5. *Cross-reference with content.* The astronomical framework provides context, not content. The phonetic and paradoxical methods of Chapter Four still apply to the dream's imagery. The hour and decan tell you *when* and *under what influence*; the image analysis tells you *what*.

## Sources


Neugebauer, Otto, and Richard A. Parker. *Egyptian Astronomical Texts.* 3 vols. Providence: Brown University Press, 1960–1969.

Leitz, Christian. *Altägyptische Sternuhren.* Leuven: Peeters, 1995.

Hornung, Erik. *The Ancient Egyptian Books of the Afterlife.* Translated by David Lorton. Ithaca: Cornell University Press, 1999.

Klotz, David. 'Dream Interpreters and Incubation at Egyptian Sanctuaries.' In *Greco-Egyptian Interactions*, edited by Ian Rutherford, 285–310. Oxford: Oxford University Press, 2016.

Spalinger, Anthony. 'Ancient Egyptian Calendars and Chronology.' In *Ancient Egyptian Chronology*, edited by Erik Hornung et al., 224–268. Leiden: Brill, 2006.

## Appendix C

# Tables of Essential Dignities

The essential dignities constitute the primary system for evaluating planetary strength in traditional astrology. A planet possessing essential dignity operates according to its own nature. In dream judgment, the essential dignity of the significator indicates the dream's potential for accurate prophecy.

## *Dorothean Triplicity Lords*

*Table C.1. Dorothean triplicity lords.*

| Triplicity | Signs | Day Lord | Night Lord | Participant |
|---|---|---|---|---|
| Fire | Aries, Leo, Sagittarius | Sun | Jupiter | Saturn |
| Earth | Taurus, Virgo, Capricorn | Venus | Moon | Mars |
| Air | Gemini, Libra, Aquarius | Saturn | Mercury | Jupiter |
| Water | Cancer, Scorpio, Pisces | Venus | Mars | Moon |

## *Complete Essential Dignities*

*Table C.2. Complete essential dignities by sign.*

| Sign | Domicile | Exaltation | Day Trip. | Night Trip. | Particip. |
|---|---|---|---|---|---|
| Aries | Mars | Sun (19°) | Sun | Jupiter | Saturn |
| Taurus | Venus | Moon (3°) | Venus | Moon | Mars |
| Gemini | Mercury | North Node | Saturn | Mercury | Jupiter |
| Cancer | Moon | Jupiter (15°) | Venus | Mars | Moon |
| Leo | Sun | — | Sun | Jupiter | Saturn |
| Virgo | Mercury | Mercury (15°) | Venus | Moon | Mars |
| Libra | Venus | Saturn (21°) | Saturn | Mercury | Jupiter |
| Scorpio | Mars | — | Venus | Mars | Moon |
| Sagittarius | Jupiter | South Node | Sun | Jupiter | Saturn |
| Capricorn | Saturn | Mars (28°) | Venus | Moon | Mars |
| Aquarius | Saturn | — | Saturn | Mercury | Jupiter |
| Pisces | Jupiter | Venus (27°) | Venus | Mars | Moon |

## Essential Dignity Point Values

For calculating the Almuten: Domicile (+5), Exaltation (+4), Triplicity (+3), Term (+2), Face (+1). Essential debilities—detriment and fall—do not subtract points but indicate a planet operating contrary to its nature.

*Table C.3. Complete essential dignities*

| Hellenistic | 1pt | 1pt | 1pt | | | 1pt | | | | | 1pt | | |
|---|---|---|---|---|---|---|---|---|---|---|---|---|---|
| Renaissance | 5pt | 4pt | 3pt | | | 2pt | | | | | 1pt | | |
| Sign | Ruler | Exalt | Triplicity | | | Terms | | | | | Faces | | |
| | | | Day | Night | Mix | | | | | | 0-10 | 10-20 | 20-30 |
| ♈ | ♂ | ☉ 19 | ☉ | ♃ | ♄ | ♃ 6 | ♀ 14 | ☿ 21 | ♂ 26 | ♄ 30 | ♂ | ☉ | ♀ |
| ♉ | ♀ | ☽ 15 | ♀ | ☽ | ♂ | ♀ 8 | ☿ 15 | ♃ 22 | ♄ 26 | ♂ 30 | ☿ | ☽ | ♄ |
| ♊ | ☿ | ☊ 3 | ♄ | ☿ | ♃ | ☿ 7 | ♃ 14 | ♀ 21 | ♄ 25 | ♂ 30 | ♃ | ♂ | ☉ |
| ♋ | ☽ | ♃ 15 | ♀♂ | ♂ | ☽ | ♂ 6 | ♃ 13 | ☿ 20 | ♀ 27 | ♄ 30 | ♀ | ☿ | ☽ |
| ♌ | ☉ | | ☉ | ♃ | ♄ | ♄ 6 | ☿ 13 | ♀ 19 | ♃ 25 | ♂ 30 | ♄ | ♃ | ♂ |
| ♍ | ☿ | ☿ 15 | ♀ | ☽ | ♂ | ☿ 7 | ♀ 13 | ♃ 18 | ♄ 24 | ♂ 30 | ☉ | ♀ | ☿ |
| ♎ | ♀ | ♄ 21 | ♄ | ☿ | ♃ | ♄ 6 | ♀ 11 | ♃ 19 | ☿ 24 | ♂ 30 | ☽ | ♄ | ♃ |
| ♏ | ♂ | | ♀♂ | ♂ | ☽ | ♂ 6 | ♃ 14 | ♀ 21 | ☿ 27 | ♄ 30 | ♂ | ☉ | ♀ |
| ♐ | ♃ | ☋ 3 | ☉ | ♃ | ♄ | ♃ 8 | ♀ 14 | ☿ 19 | ♄ 25 | ♂ 30 | ☿ | ☽ | ♄ |
| ♑ | ♄ | ♂ 28 | ♀ | ☽ | ♂ | ♀ 6 | ☿ 12 | ♃ 19 | ♂ 25 | ♄ 30 | ♃ | ♂ | ☉ |
| ♒ | ♄ | | ♄ | ☿ | ♃ | ♄ 6 | ☿ 12 | ♀ 20 | ♃ 25 | ♂ 30 | ♀ | ☿ | ☽ |
| ♓ | ♃ | ♀ 17 | ♀♂ | ♂ | ☽ | ♀ 8 | ♃ 14 | ☿ 20 | ♂ 26 | ♄ 30 | ♄ | ♃ | ♂ |

APPENDIX D

# Planetary Hours and Lunar Timing

# Planetary Hours

The planetary hours follow the Chaldean order—Saturn, Jupiter, Mars, Sun, Venus, Mercury, Moon—descending from slowest to swiftest. Each day begins at local sunrise with the hour of that day's ruler.

# Planetary Day Rulers

*Table D.1. Planetary day rulers and dream qualities.*

| Day | Ruler | Dream Qualities |
|---|---|---|
| Sunday | Sun | Authority, clarity, success, the Self; prophetic for health |
| Monday | Moon | Emotion, memory, the feminine, travel, fluctuation |
| Tuesday | Mars | Conflict, energy, passion, danger; prophetic for courage |
| Wednesday | Mercury | Communication, messages, learning; prophetic for contracts |
| Thursday | Jupiter | Expansion, religion, fortune; most favorable for prophetic dreams |
| Friday | Venus | Love, art, pleasure; prophetic for unions and beauty |
| Saturday | Saturn | Limitation, endings, ancestors; prophetic for long-term fate |

## *Calculation Method*

**Step 1.** Determine sunrise and sunset times for the location and date.

**Step 2.** Calculate diurnal hour length: (Sunset − Sunrise) ÷ 12.

**Step 3.** Calculate nocturnal hour length: (Next Sunrise − Sunset) ÷ 12.

**Step 4.** Identify which hour contains the dream time.

**Step 5.** Apply the Chaldean sequence from the day ruler.

# Diurnal Planetary Hours

*Table D.2. Diurnal planetary hours (sunrise to sunset).*

| Hour | Sunday | Monday | Tuesday | Wednesday | Thursday | Friday | Saturday |
|---|---|---|---|---|---|---|---|
| 1 | Sun | Moon | Mars | Mercury | Jupiter | Venus | Saturn |
| 2 | Venus | Saturn | Sun | Moon | Mars | Mercury | Jupiter |
| 3 | Mercury | Jupiter | Venus | Saturn | Sun | Moon | Mars |
| 4 | Moon | Mars | Mercury | Jupiter | Venus | Saturn | Sun |
| 5 | Saturn | Sun | Moon | Mars | Mercury | Jupiter | Venus |
| 6 | Jupiter | Venus | Saturn | Sun | Moon | Mars | Mercury |
| 7 | Mars | Mercury | Jupiter | Venus | Saturn | Sun | Moon |
| 8 | Sun | Moon | Mars | Mercury | Jupiter | Venus | Saturn |
| 9 | Venus | Saturn | Sun | Moon | Mars | Mercury | Jupiter |
| 10 | Mercury | Jupiter | Venus | Saturn | Sun | Moon | Mars |
| 11 | Moon | Mars | Mercury | Jupiter | Venus | Saturn | Sun |
| 12 | Saturn | Sun | Moon | Mars | Mercury | Jupiter | Venus |

## Nocturnal Planetary Hours

*Table D.3. Nocturnal planetary hours (sunset to sunrise).*

| Hour | Sun Night | Mon Night | Tue Night | Wed Night | Thu Night | Fri Night | Sat Night |
|---|---|---|---|---|---|---|---|
| 1 | Jupiter | Venus | Saturn | Sun | Moon | Mars | Mercury |
| 2 | Mars | Mercury | Jupiter | Venus | Saturn | Sun | Moon |
| 3 | Sun | Moon | Mars | Mercury | Jupiter | Venus | Saturn |
| 4 | Venus | Saturn | Sun | Moon | Mars | Mercury | Jupiter |
| 5 | Mercury | Jupiter | Venus | Saturn | Sun | Moon | Mars |
| 6 | Moon | Mars | Mercury | Jupiter | Venus | Saturn | Sun |
| 7 | Saturn | Sun | Moon | Mars | Mercury | Jupiter | Venus |
| 8 | Jupiter | Venus | Saturn | Sun | Moon | Mars | Mercury |
| 9 | Mars | Mercury | Jupiter | Venus | Saturn | Sun | Moon |
| 10 | Sun | Moon | Mars | Mercury | Jupiter | Venus | Saturn |
| 11 | Venus | Saturn | Sun | Moon | Mars | Mercury | Jupiter |
| 12 | Mercury | Jupiter | Venus | Saturn | Sun | Moon | Mars |

### *Mesopotamian Lunar Timing*

Mesopotamians divided the night into three watches (*maṣṣarāti*), each governing distinct dream quality. The monthly cycle of Sîn (the Moon) further structured dream assessment.

### *The Three Watches of the Night*

*The First Watch (Evening)*: The Watch of the People. Dreams reflect the day's residue—digestion, emotion, symptoms. Least prophetic weight.

*The Second Watch (Midnight)*: The Watch of the Gods. The soul travels deepest, entering the Central Void. Greatest spiritual significance. The *zaqīqu* is most receptive to divine transmission.

*The Third Watch (Dawn)*: The Watch of the Morning. Dreams are prescriptive—specific guidance, formulas, actions needed for healing. Often manifest quickly.

## The Lunar Month and Dream Potency

*Table D.4. Mesopotamian lunar gates and dream qualities.*

| Day | Phase | Gate | Dream Quality |
|---|---|---|---|
| 1 | *Arhu (New Crescent)* | The Portal | Emergence of Sîn. Dreams are seeding events—good for identifying roots of new pathology. |
| 7 | *Eššeššu I (First Quarter)* | The Balance | Moon half-illuminated. Dreams are diagnostic, showing tension between sick spirit and vital breath. |
| 15 | *Šapattu (Full Moon)* | The Zenith | Peak of noetic light. Dreams are mātu—true, prognostic. Night of the Divine Decree. |
| 21 | *Eššeššu II (Last Quarter)* | The Descent | Moon returns toward the void. Dreams are purgative, often involving release of ancestral debts. |
| 29/30 | *Bubbulum (Conjunction)* | The Abyss | Sîn in the Netherworld. Dreams are chthonic—prime time for communication with etêmmu (ghosts). |

## Application

Consider both watch and lunar phase. A dream received during the Second Watch on the night of *Šapattu* carries maximum prophetic weight. A First Watch dream on an ordinary night likely reflects residue rather than divine communication.

The Vedic four watches (Chapter Five) and the tripartite night in Western clinical practice (Chapter Thirteen) are parallel developments: not all hours of darkness are equal for dream reception.

## Appendix E

# Almuten Calculation and Five-Flavor Applications

The Almuten (from Arabic *al-mubtazz,* "the victor") is the planet with the greatest cumulative essential dignity at a specific zodiacal degree. This appendix guides Almuten calculation, then demonstrates application to five-flavor dream therapeutics.

## Essential Dignity Point Values

*Table E.1. Essential dignity point values.*

| Dignity | Points | Notes |
|---|---|---|
| Domicile | +5 | Strongest dignity; planet rules the sign |
| Exaltation | +4 | Elevated functioning; specific degree |
| Triplicity | +3 | Elemental affinity; consider sect |
| Term (Bound) | +2 | Rulership of degree range |
| Face (Decan) | +1 | Weakest dignity; 10-degree divisions |

## Almuten Calculation: Worked Example

Given: 9th house cusp at 15° Scorpio in a nocturnal chart.

*Table E.2. Almuten calculation for 15° Scorpio (nocturnal chart).*

| Dignity | Saturn | Jupiter | Mars | Sun | Venus | Mercury |
|---|---|---|---|---|---|---|
| Domicile (+5) | — | — | 5 | — | — | — |
| Exaltation (+4) | — | — | — | — | — | — |
| Triplicity (+3) | — | — | 3 | — | — | — |
| Term (+2) | — | 2 | — | — | — | — |
| Face (+1) | — | — | — | 1 | — | — |
| Total | 0 | 2 | 8 | 1 | 0 | 0 |

**Result:** Mars is the Almuten of 15° Scorpio with 8 points (domicile + triplicity).

# Application to Five-Flavor Dream Therapeutics

The Almuten calculation underlies the five-flavor protocol of Chapter Six. Once the practitioner identifies which planets hold dignity over a degree—whether Jupiter's position or the ninth house cusp—each visible planet contributes its corresponding organ-spirit to the assessment. The following examples demonstrate both methods in full.

## *Method One: Jupiter's Dignities*

Since the ethereal soul (*hún*) is the dream-generator, Jupiter's condition guides treatment. Cast a chart for when the dream is reported. Identify every planet ruling Jupiter's position by domicile, exaltation, triplicity, term, and face. Each visible planet contributes one herb, addressing all planetary influences on the *hún*'s condition.

Hellenistic astrologers assigned equal weight to each dignity. The weighted system (5 for domicile, 4 for exaltation, 3 for triplicity, 2 for term, 1 for face) emerged in Persian and Arabic periods. Make your choice and understand why, or use both until advantages emerge for different questions.

## *Worked Example: Jupiter at 12° Cancer (Nocturnal Chart)*

The querent asks about recurring nightmares. Horary shows Jupiter at 12° Cancer, nocturnal chart.

Identify every planet contributing dignity to Jupiter's position:

*Domicile:* Moon rules Cancer. Luminaries don't participate in the flavor protocol—no contribution.

*Exaltation:* Jupiter himself exalts in Cancer. Wood/Liver/*hún*.

*Triplicity:* Cancer belongs to the Water triplicity. At night, Mars rules; Venus participates. Mars contributes Fire/Heart/*shén*. Venus contributes Metal/Lung/*pò*.

*Term:* At 12° Cancer, Mercury rules the term. Water/Kidney/*zhì*.

*Face:* Mercury also rules the face but is already counted.

Four visible planets contribute dignity: Jupiter (exaltation), Mars and Venus (triplicity), Mercury (term). Four planets, four organ-spirits to address.

*Table E.3. Dignity calculation for Jupiter at 12° Cancer (nocturnal chart).*

| Dignity | Ruler | Visible? | Contribution |
|---|---|---|---|
| Domicile | Moon | No | — |
| Exaltation | Jupiter | Yes | Wood/Liver/hún |
| Triplicity (night) | Mars, Venus | Yes | Fire/Heart/shén; Metal/Lung/pò |
| Term | Mercury | Yes | Water/Kidney/zhì |
| Face | Mercury | Yes | (already counted) |

## *Determining the Therapeutic Action*

Jupiter in Cancer holds exaltation—strongly dignified. The *hún* functions robustly; supplementation unnecessary. The querent reports excessive dreaming, vivid imagery that exhausts rather than restores, stress upon waking. Excess activity of the ethereal soul requiring reduction. From Table 6.4: for Jupiter (Wood/Liver/*hún*), sour reduces.

## *Kitchen Practice*

Reducing action calls for sour flavor across all four organ systems. Build meals around this principle for one lunar cycle or until dream quality shifts.

*Morning:* Start with warm water and lemon. Breakfast congee with pickled vegetables and a splash of black vinegar.

*Midday:* Salad of bitter greens (arugula, dandelion, radicchio) dressed with citrus vinaigrette. The bitter supports Mercury/Kidney/*zhì* while the citrus maintains the sour emphasis. Add fermented vegetables—sauerkraut, kimchi, or quick-pickled radish.

*Evening:* The main therapeutic meal.

# Sour Broth with Poached Fish and Seasonal Vegetables

Bring four cups of water to a simmer with two tablespoons of rice vinegar, one tablespoon of tamari, a thumb of sliced ginger, and three dried shiitake mushrooms. Let steep twenty minutes. Remove ginger and mushrooms, slice mushrooms thin, return to broth. Add one cup of leafy greens (bok choy, spinach, or watercress for Metal/Lung/*pò*), half cup of cubed winter squash or sweet potato (for Earth/Spleen, grounding the formula), and a handful of wood ear mushrooms (for Wood/Liver/*hún*). Simmer until vegetables soften. Poach four ounces of white fish (cod, sole, or sea bass) in the broth until just cooked through. Finish with another splash of rice vinegar, a squeeze of lime, and a scattering of fresh cilantro. Serve with a small dish of pickled plums on the side.

The sourness pervades. Each organ-spirit receives the reducing message through flavor. Vinegar in the broth addresses Liver/*hún* directly. The fish and tamari carry the salty undercurrent supporting Kidney/*zhì*. Leafy greens and the astringent quality of citrus address Lung/*pò*. The broth's warmth and the sweet potato provide just enough Earth to ground the formula.

*Evening tea:* Schisandra berry infusion. Five-flavor berry, but sour predominates. Steep one tablespoon of dried berries in hot water for ten minutes. Drink before bed.

Consistency matters more than quantity. The medicinal kitchen works through repetition—daily flavor emphasis accumulating over weeks, redirecting organ-spirits toward balance. When dream quality improves, ease off sour emphasis and return to varied eating.

## *Method Two: The Term Ruler of the Ninth Cusp*

A more direct method focuses on the term ruler of the ninth house cusp. Since terms divide each sign into five segments ruled by different planets, the term ruler indicates which organ-spirit most immediately shapes prophetic access.

# Worked Example: Ninth Cusp at 22° Virgo

The querent asks why dreams feel muddled, repetitive, impossible to interpret. Ninth cusp at 22° Virgo.

In Virgo, terms are distributed as follows: Mercury to 7°, Venus to 13°, Jupiter to 18°, Saturn to 24°, Mars to 30°. At 22°, Saturn holds the term.

*Table E.4. Egyptian terms for Virgo.*

| Degrees | Term Ruler | Organ-Spirit |
| --- | --- | --- |
| 0°–7° | Mercury | Water/Kidney/zhì |
| 7°–13° | Venus | Metal/Lung/pò |
| 13°–18° | Jupiter | Wood/Liver/hún |
| 18°–24° | Saturn | Earth/Spleen/yì |
| 24°–30° | Mars | Fire/Heart/shén |

Saturn corresponds to Earth, the Spleen, and the *yì*—the organ-spirit governing intellect, concentration, the capacity to transform thought into action. When the *yì* is compromised, the mind circles without landing. Thoughts repeat. Meaning slips away. The querent's complaint—muddled imagery, repetitive cycles, inability to extract meaning—matches the pattern exactly. The term ruler has identified the organ-spirit shaping this dreamer's difficulty.

Now assess Jupiter. If Jupiter holds essential dignity, the *hún* functions adequately and treatment targets the Spleen directly. If Jupiter is peregrine or debilitated, address both. In this chart, Jupiter occupies 8° Sagittarius—his own domicile, strongly dignified. The dream-generator is robust. Treatment focuses on Saturn/Spleen/*yì*.

From Table 6.4: for Saturn (Earth/Spleen/*yì*), bitter transforms, aromatic reduces, sweet supplements. The querent's dreams are heavy, sinking, stuck in loops—a deficiency pattern, not excess. Sweet supplements.

### *Kitchen Practice*

Build meals around the full, nourishing sweetness of whole foods—not sugar, but the deep sweetness of slow-cooked grains, root vegetables, and long-simmered broths. This is Earth medicine: grounding, centering, substantial.

*Morning:* Steel-cut oats cooked slowly with cinnamon, topped with stewed apples and a drizzle of honey. The sweetness should feel sustaining, not cloying.

*Midday:* Roasted root vegetables—sweet potato, parsnip, carrot, beet—dressed lightly with olive oil and a pinch of sea salt. A cup of bone broth on the side.

*Evening:* The main therapeutic meal.

## Long-Simmered Chicken and Root Vegetable Stew

Place one whole chicken (or four bone-in thighs) in a heavy pot with eight cups of water. Add one onion quartered, four cloves of garlic, a thumb of ginger sliced, and a four-inch piece of astragalus root if available. Bring to a boil, skim, and reduce to a bare simmer. Cook for three hours. Remove chicken, strip meat, discard bones. Strain broth. Return broth to the pot with the chicken meat. Add two cups of cubed butternut squash, one cup of diced sweet potato, one cup of sliced shiitake mushrooms, and a handful of goji berries. Simmer until vegetables are tender. Season with tamari and a teaspoon of rice wine. Serve over rice with a few drops of toasted sesame oil.

The sweetness here is cumulative—from the long cooking, from the root vegetables, from the berries. Nothing sharp. Nothing sour. The *yì* needs steadiness, substance, support. Avoid raw foods, cold drinks, and excessive thinking during meals. Eat slowly. Chew thoroughly. Let the Spleen do its work.

*Evening tea:* Licorice root infusion. Steep a few slices of dried licorice in hot water for ten minutes. Mildly sweet, deeply grounding.

Continue for one lunar cycle. When dreams begin to clarify—when meaning emerges and repetition fades—the *yì* is strengthening. Ease back into varied eating while maintaining the sweet foundation.

## Dosage and Timing

Spirit doses—drop doses of tincture, pinch doses of powder—suffice for soul-level treatment. Power lies in coherence, not quantity. Administer during planetary hours aligned with intention. For *hún*-level treatment, use Jupiter hours. For dream quality specifically, the hour of the ninth house ruler. When addressing a specific planet's influence on the *hún*, use that planet's hour.

## Appendix F

# Arudha Lagna Calculation

The *Arudha Lagna* (AL) represents projected image—how one appears to others. In Jaimini astrology, dreams often reveal discrepancies between self-perception and projected image.

## Calculation Method

Step 1. Identify the Ascendant lord (1st house ruler).

Step 2. Count signs from Ascendant to the 1st lord's house.

Step 3. Count same number forward from the 1st lord's position.

Step 4. Result is the Arudha Lagna.

*Exception:* If arudha falls in 1st or 7th from original house, move to 10th sign.

## Worked Example

*Given:* Aries Ascendant. Mars (1st lord) in Gemini (3rd house).

Step 1: 1st lord = Mars

Step 2: Aries to Gemini = 3 signs

Step 3: Gemini + 3 signs = Leo

Step 4: Leo is not 1st or 7th from Aries, so Arudha Lagna

## Part II: Therapeutic Protocols

### Appendix G

# The Neurochemical Architecture of Dreaming

This appendix presents contemporary neuroscientific understanding of dream generation. The purpose is not reduction but bridge-building between traditional frameworks and modern pharmacology. Planetary correspondences proposed here represent heuristic pattern, not established mechanism—invitations to refinement through practice, not doctrine.

# I. Sleep Molecules

*Adenosine (Saturn): The Sleep Debt.* Adenosine accumulates during waking hours, producing sleepiness—pressure building until payment comes due. Caffeine blocks adenosine receptors without eliminating the debt. Extended caffeine use followed by withdrawal produces adenosine rebound, often accompanied by unusually vivid dreaming.

*GABA (Venus-Moon) and Glutamate (Mars-Sun): The On/Off Switch.* Sleep involves shift between glutamate (excitatory, Mars-Sun) and GABA (inhibitory, Venus-Moon). Benzodiazepines and alcohol enhance GABA activity; while promoting sleep onset, both suppress REM sleep.

*Melatonin (Sun-Moon-Neptune): The Circadian Orchestrator.* Melatonin, secreted by the pineal in response to darkness, does not induce sleep but serves as circadian timekeeper. The pineal responds to the Sun's absence rather than its presence—the circadian clock operating through Sun-Moon polarity.

# II. The Dream Engine: REM Neurochemistry

*Acetylcholine (Mercury-Neptune): The Dream Conductor.* Acetylcholine plays the central role in REM generation, driving vivid hallucinatory imagery. Substances enhancing cholinergic transmission—galantamine, rivastigmine, donepezil—consistently increase dream vividness and recall.

*Norepinephrine and Serotonin (Mars, Sun): The Monoamine Pause.* During REM, the locus coeruleus (norepinephrine, Mars) and raphe nuclei (serotonin, Sun) fall nearly silent. This withdrawal explains why dreamers accept impossible scenarios.

*Dopamine (Jupiter-Sun): Narrative Drive and Salience.* Dopamine drives salience marking and narrative construction—the meaning-making function suggesting Jupiter-Sun correspondence: expansion, coherence, the weaving of significance.

# III. Pharmacological Modifiers

*REM Rebound.* When REM is suppressed—by alcohol, cannabis, benzodiazepines, or antidepressants—the brain compensates upon withdrawal with prolonged, intensified REM periods and unusually vivid, often disturbing dreams.

*Galantamine and Lucid Dreaming.* Galantamine, an acetylcholinesterase inhibitor, has become the pharmacological cornerstone of lucid dreaming. Taken during a middle-of-night awakening (4–8 mg after 5 hours of sleep), it enhances cholinergic tone during the subsequent REM period.

# IV. Summary of Correspondences

*Table G.1. Neurochemistry and planetary rulers.*

| Molecule | Function | Proposed Ruler |
|---|---|---|
| Adenosine | Sleep debt, accumulation | Saturn |
| GABA | Inhibition, the switch | Venus-Moon |
| Glutamate | Excitation, waking | Mars-Sun |
| Acetylcholine | Vivid REM, hallucination | Mercury-Neptune |
| Dopamine | Narrative drive, salience | Jupiter-Sun |
| Norepinephrine | Alertness, memory | Mars |
| Melatonin | Circadian rhythm, darkness | Sun-Moon-Neptune |

Appendix H

# Oneirobotanical Comparative Materia Medica

Appendix G presented neurochemical architecture in contemporary terms. This appendix bridges that framework with celestial medicine. The synthesis is not reductive: we do not claim that "Moon" simply means "GABA antagonism." Rather, two epistemologies converge on consistent patterns.

# The Sky Medicine Matrix

*Table H.1. Sky Medicine Matrix: Neuro-cosmological Correspondences*

| Ruler | Plant | Function | Mechanism | Dream Effect |
|---|---|---|---|---|
| ☽ | *Artemisiae Vulgaris Hb.* (Mugwort) | Opens gates | GABA antagonism (thujone) | Maintains awareness in REM |
| ☽ ♄ | *Salsolae Herba* (Maštakal) | Purification | Alkaline saponins; olfactory-limbic | Cleanses nightmare residue |
| ☉ | *Lauri Nobilis Fol.* (Bay Laurel) | Illuminates symbols | Cineole (monoterpene) | Renders imagery intelligible |
| ☿ | *Celastri Paniculati Sem.* (Intellect Tree) | Enhances recall | Cholinergic potentiation | Increases vividness |
| ☿ | *Polygalae Tenuifoliae Rad.* (Polygala) | Opens orifices | Triterpenoid saponins; cholinergic | Enhances lucidity |
| ☿ | *Lavandulae Angustifoliae Fl.* (Lavender) | Calms spirit | Linalool; GABAergic | Reduces nightmare frequency |
| ♀ | *Nymphaeae Caeruleae Fl.* (Blue Lotus) | Opens the heart | Aporphine; dopaminergic | Enhances narrative salience |
| ♃ ☿ | *Caleae Zacatechichi Fol.* (Dream Herb) | Prophetic visions | Sesquiterpene lactones | Increases prophetic clarity |
| ♃ | *Ziziphi Spinosae Sem.* (Sour Jujube) | Nourishes Heart | Jujubosides; GABAergic | Reduces disturbed dreaming |

| Ruler | Plant | Function | Mechanism | Dream Effect |
|---|---|---|---|---|
| ♄ | *Mandragorae Rad.* (Mandrake) | Fate-cutter | Tropane; anticholinergic | Suppresses REM; threshold state |
| ♄ | *Silenes Capensis Rad.* (African Dream Root) | Ancestor contact | Triterpenoid saponins | Enhances ancestral dreams |
| ♄ ♂ | *Withaniae Somniferae Rad.* (Ashwagandha) | Restores substrate | Withanolides; adaptogenic | Normalizes sleep |
| ☉ ♃ ♄ | *Ginseng Rad.* (Ginseng) | Restores qì | Ginsenosides; multiple targets | Supports dream substrate |

# I. The Cholinergic Engine: Moon and Mercury

Moon governs gates and permeability. Mercury governs communication and memory. Together they preside over the cholinergic system driving REM. Mugwort (*Artemisia vulgaris* L.), ruled by the Moon, operates through GABA antagonism, maintaining presence during REM.

# II. The Dopaminergic Salience: Venus

Venus governs desire, beauty, the sense that something matters—qualities mapped onto dopamine's role in salience. Blue Lotus (*Nymphaea caerulea* Savigny) contains aporphine alkaloids with dopamine receptor affinity. Venus makes the dream feel important.

# III. The Anticholinergic Void: Saturn

Saturn rules thresholds between worlds. Mandrake (*Mandragora officinarum* L.) contains tropane alkaloids producing profound anticholinergic effects: REM suppression, altered perception, liminal states where ancestral contact becomes possible. This is not dream enhancement but dream transformation.

# IV. Substrate Restoration: The Hún and Shén Axis

Dreams require a substrate—the *hún* (ethereal soul) rooted in Liver blood and the *shén* (spirit) housed in the Heart. When depleted, dreams become disturbed or absent. Restoration of substrate may be more important than direct dream enhancement.

*Table H.2. Substrate Restoration Plants*

| Plant | Ruler | CCM Action | Biochemistry | Use |
|---|---|---|---|---|
| *Ziziphi Spinosae Sem.* (*suān zǎo rén*) | ♃ | Nourishes Heart yin | Jujubosides; GABAergic | Insomnia, anxiety |
| *Polygalae Tenuifoliae Rad.* (*yuǎn zhì*) | ☿ | Opens orifices, calms spirit | Triterpenoid saponins | Cognitive decline |
| *Withaniae Somniferae Rad.* (Ashwagandha) | ♄ ♂ | Strengthens vitality | Withanolides; adaptogenic | Chronic fatigue |
| *Ginseng Rad.* (*rén shēn*) | ☉ ♃ ♄ | Tonifies qì | Ginsenosides; nootropic | Exhaustion |

# V. Convergence and Divergence

These correspondences are not coincidences but convergent discoveries—traditional observers cataloguing effects over centuries, modern pharmacologists identifying mechanisms over decades. Yet planetary rulership captures qualities pharmacology misses: the meaning of a Venus dream, the weight of Saturn's intervention, the illumination of solar clarity. The practitioner who understands both possesses tools neither tradition alone provides.

Appendix I

# Persian-Arabic Dream Methods

This appendix provides operational procedures for Persian and Arabic methods from Chapter Eleven. These techniques complement Hellenistic methods (Chapter Ten) and Bonatti's protocols (Chapter Twelve) with timing refinements, classification filters, and ethical guidelines specific to the Islamic and Zoroastrian transmission.

# I. The Threefold Classification

Before applying interpretive technique, classify the dream. Not all dreams warrant prophetic interpretation. The Islamic tradition provides a robust first-pass filter.

## *Decision Tree (see table G.1. for Persian terms*

1. Did the dream occur in the fourth watch (approximately 3 AM to dawn)?

   If no → more likely *ḥadīth al-nafs* (psychological processing) or *ḥulm* (disturbing). If yes → continue.

2. Did the dreamer wake directly to the day without returning to sleep?

   If no → prophetic charge may have dissipated (parallels Vedic 'broken dream' principle). If yes → continue.

3. Does the dream leave a lasting, solemn impression?

   If no → likely *ḥadīth al-nafs*. If yes → continue.

4. Is the dream internally coherent with clear narrative structure?

   If no (jumbled, fragmented, fearful) → likely *ḥulm*. Protective response indicated. If yes → continue.

5. Does the content concern matters beyond the dreamer's ordinary knowledge?

   If no → may be *ḥadīth al-nafs* reflecting daily concerns. If yes → likely *ru'ya* (true dream). Proceed to interpretation.

*Table I.1: Classification Summary*

| Type | Characteristics | Source | Response |
|---|---|---|---|
| Ru'ya | Fourth watch; coherent; lasting impression; novel content | Divine/angelic communication | Interpret prophetically |
| Ḥulm | Disturbing; fragmented; fearful; confusing | Demonic interference | Protective measures; do not interpret |
| Ḥadīth al-nafs | Reflects daily concerns; bodily states; anxieties | Psychological processing | Recognize source; no prophetic weight |

### *Protective Response for Ḥulm*

When a dream is classified as *ḥulm* (disturbing/demonic):

1. Do not recount the dream to others (recounting may 'ground' negative content).
2. Spit lightly three times to the left upon waking.
3. Seek refuge through prayer or protective mantra appropriate to the dreamer's tradition.
4. Change sleeping position if returning to sleep.
5. Give charitable offering the following day to redirect the energy.

## II. Firdaria: Life Chapters for Dream Interpretation

The *firdaria* divides life into planetary chapters. Dream significance is modified by which planet rules the current chapter.

### *Step 1: Determine Sect*

Was the native born by day (Sun above horizon) or night (Sun below)?

Day birth → Diurnal sequence (begins with Sun)

Night birth → Nocturnal sequence (begins with Moon)

*Table I.2: Step 2, Identify Current Major Period*

| Planet | Years | Diurnal Ages | Nocturnal Ages |
|---|---|---|---|
| Sun | 10 | 0–10 | 39–49 |
| Venus | 8 | 10–18 | 49–57 |
| Mercury | 13 | 18–31 | 57–70 |
| Moon | 9 | 31–40 | 0–9 |
| Saturn | 11 | 40–51 | 9–20 |
| Jupiter | 12 | 51–63 | 20–32 |
| Mars | 7 | 63–70 | 32–39 |
| North Node | 3 | 70–73 | 70–73 |
| South Node | 2 | 73–75 | 73–75 |

## *Step 3: Calculate Sub-Period (Optional)*

Each major period divides into seven sub-periods of equal length. The first sub-period is ruled by the major period ruler; subsequent sub-periods follow Chaldean order (Saturn → Jupiter → Mars → Sun → Venus → Mercury → Moon).

Sub-period length = Major period years ÷ 7

Example: Saturn major period (11 years) → sub-periods of approximately 1 year, 7 months each.

*Table I.3: Step 4: Apply to Dream Interpretation*

| Firdar Lord | Dream Themes Emphasized | Interpretive Guidance |
|---|---|---|
| Sun | Authority, identity, father, vitality, public role | Dreams may address core purpose; literal fulfillment more likely |
| Moon | Emotions, mother, home, body, the public | Heightened dream receptivity; emotional content amplified |
| Mercury | Communication, siblings, commerce, learning | Message-dreams common; symbolic content requires careful decoding |

| Firdar Lord | Dream Themes Emphasized | Interpretive Guidance |
|---|---|---|
| Venus | Relationships, pleasure, art, values, women | 'Sweet dreams'; relational content; aesthetic imagery |
| Mars | Conflict, surgery, fever, brothers, action | Aggressive imagery more common; may reflect necessary action |
| Jupiter | Expansion, wisdom, teachers, religion, wealth | Prophetic dreams more likely; benefic content; guidance figures |
| Saturn | Restriction, elders, death, karma, structure | Heavy dreams addressing duty; ancestral themes; endings |
| North Node | Increase, obsession, foreign influences | Amplification; desires; disorienting content |
| South Node | Decrease, release, spirituality, loss | Dreams of letting go; past-life themes; mokṣa content |

## *Step 5: Assess Firdar Lord's Natal Condition*

The natal condition of the current *firdar* lord determines whether the chapter—and dreams within it—tend toward benefit or difficulty:

**Dignified** (domicile, exaltation, triplicity): The planet can deliver its significations constructively. Dreams during this period more likely to be *ru'ya* with positive outcomes.

**Debilitated** (detriment, fall): The planet struggles to deliver its significations. Dreams may be more troubled; careful interpretation required.

**Angular** (1st, 4th, 7th, 10th houses): The planet has power to manifest. Dreams more likely to produce concrete results.

**Cadent** (3rd, 6th, 9th, 12th houses): The planet has less power to manifest. Dreams may be vivid but less consequential.

# III. The Lord of the Turn and the Turning of the Soul

This technique identifies seven-year thresholds when the dream channel opens and transformative visions become more likely.

## *Step 1: Determine the Planetary Hour of Birth*

Planetary hour of birth requires accurate birth time. The day is divided into twelve diurnal hours (sunrise to sunset) and twelve nocturnal hours (sunset to sunrise). Each hour is ruled by a planet in Chaldean order, beginning with the day ruler.

*Table I.4 Day Rulers*

| Day | Day Ruler (1st Hour after Sunrise) |
|---|---|
| Sunday | Sun |
| Monday | Moon |
| Tuesday | Mars |
| Wednesday | Mercury |
| Thursday | Jupiter |
| Friday | Venus |
| Saturday | Saturn |

Subsequent hours follow Chaldean order: Saturn → Jupiter → Mars → Sun → Venus → Mercury → Moon → Saturn...

Calculate which hour contains the birth time. That planet is the Lord of the Turn for year one of life.

## *Step 2: Assign Lords to Subsequent Years*

Each year of life is ruled by the next planet in Chaldean sequence:

Year 1: Birth-hour planet

Year 2: Next in Chaldean order

Year 3: Next in Chaldean order

...and so on, cycling through all seven planets every seven years.

## *Step 3: Identify the Turning of the Soul*

The specific 'Turning of the Soul' occurs when the Lord of the Turn coincides with the lord of the Moon's natal nakṣatra (lunar mansion). This requires:

1. Identify the Moon's natal nakṣatra (see Appendix J for nakṣatra tables).
2. Identify the planetary lord of that nakṣatra.
3. Note all years when the Lord of the Turn matches the nakṣatra lord.

These years are peak windows for transformative dreams—ecstatic visions, encounters with guiding figures, dreams of death and rebirth, departure from the body.

## *Example Calculation*

Native born Thursday at 3:00 PM (approximately 9th diurnal hour).

Thursday's 1st hour = Jupiter. Following Chaldean order: hour 2 = Mars, hour 3 = Sun, hour 4 = Venus, hour 5 = Mercury, hour 6 = Moon, hour 7 = Saturn, hour 8 = Jupiter, hour 9 = Mars.

Birth-hour planet = Mars. Lord of the Turn for year 1 = Mars.

Year 2 = Sun, Year 3 = Venus, Year 4 = Mercury, Year 5 = Moon, Year 6 = Saturn, Year 7 = Jupiter, Year 8 = Mars (cycle repeats).

If the natal Moon is in Mṛgaśirā nakṣatra (ruled by Mars), the Turnings of the Soul occur at ages 1, 8, 15, 22, 29, 36, 43, 50... when Mars is Lord of the Turn.

# IV. Annual Profections for Dream Interpretation

Profections rotate the chart one sign per year from the Ascendant. This ancient Hellenistic technique identifies which house—and therefore which life domain—is activated during any given year. For dream interpretation, profections reveal whether the current year emphasizes prophetic access (ninth house) or hidden disturbance (twelfth house), and identify the Lord of the Year whose condition shapes dream quality.

## *Step 1: Calculate the Profected House*

At birth (age 0), the first house is activated. Each birthday advances the profection one house. The cycle repeats every twelve years.

Age 0, 12, 24, 36, 48, 60, 72: First house (identity, body, self-presentation)

Age 1, 13, 25, 37, 49, 61, 73: Second house (resources, values, sustenance)

Age 2, 14, 26, 38, 50, 62, 74: Third house (siblings, communication, short journeys)

Age 3, 15, 27, 39, 51, 63, 75: Fourth house (home, father, foundations, endings)

Age 4, 16, 28, 40, 52, 64, 76: Fifth house (children, pleasure, creativity)

Age 5, 17, 29, 41, 53, 65, 77: Sixth house (illness, service, daily labor)

Age 6, 18, 30, 42, 54, 66, 78: Seventh house (marriage, partnerships, open enemies)

Age 7, 19, 31, 43, 55, 67, 79: Eighth house (death, inheritance, others' resources)

**Age 8, 20, 32, 44, 56, 68, 80: Ninth house (prophecy, dreams, higher knowledge, long journeys)**

Age 9, 21, 33, 45, 57, 69, 81: Tenth house (career, reputation, public action)

Age 10, 22, 34, 46, 58, 70, 82: Eleventh house (friends, hopes, benefactors)

Age 11, 23, 35, 47, 59, 71, 83: Twelfth house (hidden enemies, confinement, self-undoing)

### *Step 2: Identify the Lord of the Year*

The planet ruling the sign on the profected house cusp becomes Lord of the Year. This planet's natal condition—dignity, house placement, aspects—determines whether the year tends toward benefit or difficulty. The Lord of the Year also becomes the primary significator for dreams during that year.

Example: Native has Aries rising. At age 32, the profection reaches the ninth house (Sagittarius). Jupiter rules Sagittarius, so Jupiter is Lord of the Year. Jupiter's natal condition shapes the year's dream quality and prophetic access.

### *Step 3: Apply to Dream Interpretation*

**Ninth-house profection years** (ages 8, 20, 32, 44, 56, 68, 80) activate the *Domus Dei*—the house of prophecy, divine communication, and true dreams. During these years, the native experiences heightened dream activity, clearer prophetic content, and greater access to the *theos* dimension. Dreams occurring during ninth-house years merit more serious attention as potential *ru'ya*.

**Twelfth-house profection years** (ages 11, 23, 35, 47, 59, 71, 83) activate the house of hidden disturbance. Dreams during these years often reflect shadow material, hidden fears, unresolved grief, or unconscious patterns seeking integration. A malefic ruling the twelfth intensifies this tendency. These dreams may be psychologically significant even when not prophetically valid—the *ḥadīth al-nafs* (self-talk) category deserves attention during twelfth-house years.

**Eighth-house profection years** (ages 7, 19, 31, 43, 55, 67, 79) activate themes of death, transformation, and others' resources. Dreams of the dead, encounters with ancestors, *nigredo* imagery, and intimations of mortality are more common during these years. The alchemical staging discussed in Chapter Thirteen should be applied with particular attention.

## *Integration with Firdaria*

Profections and *firdaria* operate at different temporal scales. *Firdaria* establishes the "chapter theme" spanning years or decades; profections identify the activated house within each year. When both systems converge on dream-relevant houses, dream activity intensifies significantly.

Example: A nocturnal native at age 20 experiences Moon *firdar* (heightened dream receptivity) simultaneous with ninth-house profection (prophetic house activated). This double emphasis creates a peak window for significant dreams. If the natal Moon also occupies the ninth house or aspects its ruler, the convergence strengthens further.

## *Worked Example*

Native: Cancer rising, born during the day, currently age 44.

**Step 1:** Age 44 = ninth-house profection year. The ninth house from Cancer is Pisces.

**Step 2:** Jupiter rules Pisces. Jupiter is Lord of the Year. Check Jupiter's natal condition: assume Jupiter is in Sagittarius (own domicile) in the sixth house, trine Moon.

**Step 3:** Assessment: Ninth-house profection indicates heightened prophetic access this year. Jupiter dignified in domicile suggests the prophetic channel operates constructively. Sixth-house placement: dreams may relate to health, service, or daily work. Trine to Moon: emotional clarity in dream reception. Current *firdar* (diurnal age 44 = Saturn *firdar*): Dreams during this year likely address duty, structure, ancestral patterns, and karmic weight—but the ninth-house profection ensures prophetic validity remains high. Significant dreams this year should be taken seriously and may guide decisions about responsibility and long-term structure.

# V. Lunar Impediments Checklist

The Moon's condition in the dream chart (or natal chart) determines clarity and reliability of the dream channel. Use this checklist to assess lunar impediment.

*Table I.5 Lunar Impediments*

| Impediment | Definition | Dream Implication |
|---|---|---|
| Combust | Within 15° of Sun (applying) or 12° (separating) | Message hidden or overwhelmed |
| Under the Beams | Within 17° of Sun but not combust | Message weakened but present |
| Void of Course | Makes no major aspect before leaving sign | 'Feral' dream; nothing comes of it |
| Via Combusta | Between 15° Libra and 15° Scorpio | Extreme instability; unreliable |
| Besieged | Between Mars and Saturn by degree | Soul under attack; likely ḥulm |
| In Fall | Moon in Scorpio | Diminished receptivity |
| In Detriment | Moon in Capricorn | Cold, restricted dream content |
| Slow in Course | Less than 12° daily motion | Delayed manifestation |
| Decreasing in Light | Waning (after Full Moon) | Reflective rather than manifestive |
| In 6th, 8th, or 12th | Moon in these houses | Dream may reflect illness, crisis, or hidden matters |
| Afflicted by Malefic | Hard aspect from Mars or Saturn | Dream content colored by malefic themes |
| Conjunct South Node | Within 5° of Ketu | Spiritual/release themes; past-life content |
| Conjunct North Node | Within 5° of Rāhu | Amplified, possibly obsessive content |

### *Assessment Protocol*

Count the number of impediments affecting the Moon:

0–1 impediments: Moon is clear. Dream channel is open. Greater weight for prophetic interpretation.

2–3 impediments: Moon is moderately afflicted. Interpret with caution; consider *ḥadīth al-nafs* more likely than *ru'ya*.

4+ impediments: Moon is severely afflicted. Dream likely reflects disturbance rather than prophecy. Focus on source identification rather than predictive interpretation.

### *Benefic Mitigations*

Impediments may be mitigated by:

- Moon in domicile (Cancer) or exaltation (Taurus)
- Moon in mutual reception with a benefic
- Moon applying to trine or sextile with Jupiter or Venus
- Moon in the 9th house (place of true dreams)

## VI. Lot of Dreams Calculation

The Lot of Dreams (*Pars Somniorum*) identifies a sensitive point related to dream capacity and nocturnal communication.

### *Formula*

**Lot of Dreams = Ascendant + Mercury − Lord of the 9th House**

(If the result exceeds 360°, subtract 360°. If negative, add 360°.)

## Rationale

Mercury is messenger of the gods—translator of divine communication. The ninth house lord governs prophecy and divine dreams. Their relationship, projected from the Ascendant, indicates how effectively the native receives dream messages.

## Step-by-Step Calculation

1. Identify the Ascendant degree (e.g., 15° Aries = 15°).
2. Identify Mercury's degree in absolute longitude (Aries 0° = 0°, Taurus 0° = 30°, Gemini 0° = 60°, etc.).
3. Identify the lord of the 9th house and its degree in absolute longitude.
4. Calculate: Ascendant + Mercury − 9th Lord.
5. Convert result back to sign and degree.

## Example

- Ascendant: 15° Leo = 135° (Leo begins at 120°)
- Mercury: 22° Virgo = 172° (Virgo begins at 150°)
- 9th House: Aries. Lord = Mars. Mars at 8° Capricorn = 278° (Capricorn begins at 270°)
- Calculation: 135 + 172 − 278 = 29°
- 29° = 29° Aries
- The Lot of Dreams falls at 29° Aries.

*Table I.6 Interpretation*

| Lot Placement | Interpretation |
|---|---|
| Angular (1, 4, 7, 10) | Dreams carry weight; tend toward manifestation; native is a 'dreamer' in the prophetic sense |
| Succedent (2, 5, 8, 11) | Dreams have moderate power; may require effort to manifest or interpret |
| Cadent (3, 6, 9, 12) | Dreams vivid but less consequential; mental/spiritual significance over material |
| Conjunct benefic | Dreams tend toward positive content and outcomes |
| Conjunct malefic | Dreams may be troubling but potentially instructive; warnings common |
| In 9th house | Strong prophetic capacity; dreams as primary spiritual channel |
| In 12th house | Dreams reflect hidden material, fears, or spiritual retreat; may indicate sleep disturbances |

The condition of the Lot's dispositor (the planet ruling the sign where the Lot falls) further refines interpretation. A well-dignified dispositor supports clear, reliable dreams. An afflicted dispositor suggests the dream channel is obstructed or distorted.

# VII. The Ethics of Interpretation

Ibn Sīrīn's teaching that interpretation participates in manifestation carries practical implications.

## *Principles*

1. The dream is 'on the wing of a bird' until interpreted. The interpreter's framing helps determine how the dream grounds into reality. This is power; it demands responsibility.
2. Multiple true framings may exist. The teeth-falling dream can truthfully be framed as 'your family will die before you' or 'you will outlive your family—blessed with long life.' Both are accurate. Choose the framing that serves the dreamer's flourishing while remaining honest.

3. Silence is sometimes appropriate. Ibn Sīrīn often refused to interpret dreams he felt would ground negative outcomes. Not every dream requires interpretation. Some are better left unspoken.
4. Know when protective response supersedes interpretation. A *ḥulm* requires protection, not analysis. Interpreting demonic content may give it power. Redirect to protective measures.
5. The dreamer's state shapes meaning. The same symbol means differently for different dreamers. Assessment of spiritual/psychological condition is not optional but essential to accurate interpretation.
6. Interpretation is a religious act. Ibn Sīrīn warned: 'Look well from whom you take your religion.' The dream interpreter stands between the dreamer and the unseen. This position requires integrity, humility, and care.

## Practical Application

When interpreting a dream:

- Begin with classification (*ru'ya*/*ḥulm*/*ḥadīth al-nafs*).
- Assess celestial context (*firdaria*, lunar condition, Lot of Dreams).
- Consider the dreamer's circumstances, character, and spiritual state.
- Identify multiple possible framings before speaking.
- Choose the framing that is both true and constructive.
- If uncertain, err toward silence or toward the more benefic interpretation.
- Remember: you are participating in what the dream becomes.

APPENDIX J

# Naksatra Mantras for Sleep and Dreaming

In Vedic practice, there is no separate set of 'sleep-only' seed syllables (beeja mantras) for each naksatra; rather, traditional beeja mantras align consciousness with specific lunar energy. When applied to sleep or dreaming, these syllables 'seal' the mind into the frequency of the naksatra the Moon is transiting, or the naksatra of the twelfth house cusp.

Primary seed syllables for the twenty-seven nakṣatras appear in Table H.1. For sleep or dreaming, chant mentally (manasa japa) while drifting off, focusing on resonance rather than vocalization. In Vedic astrology and Atharva Veda traditions, specific mantras focus on sleep (*nidrā*) and dreaming (*svapna*). While every nakṣatra has a deity mantra, some align more with the subconscious and nocturnal transition.

## The Naksatra Suktam

The Nakṣatra Sūktam (Atharva Veda) contains verses for all twenty-seven constellations. Two are cited for calming influence before sleep.

Rohini (the Star of Ascent) is ruled by Prajapati the Creator. Its energy governs growth and fertility, but it is also the favorite mansion of the Moon. Chanting the Rohini mantra brings calmness and auspiciousness to the mind.

*Om Prajapataye Namah*

Anuradha (the Star of Success) is ruled by Mitra the Friend. Associated with the lotus and the ability to find harmony within, it fosters inner peace and emotional balance before rest.

*Om Mitraya Namah*

or

*Om Tam Tham Dam Anuradhayai Namah*

# Dedicated Mantras for Sleep and Dreaming

Beyond nakṣatra lords, Vedic tradition employs targeted mantras for sleep or lucid dreaming.

Nidra Devi Mantra (for deep sleep) invokes the Goddess of Sleep to ensure uninterrupted rest.

> *Ya Devi Sarva Bhutesu Nidra Rupena Samsthita Namastasyai Namastasyai Namastasyai Namo Namah*

(Salutations to the Divine Feminine who resides in all beings in the form of sleep.)

Svapnesvari Mantra (for dreaming and lucid dreaming) invokes the deity of dreams to gain clarity, answers, or awareness within the dream state.

> *Om Krim Krim Krim Hrim Hrim Svapnesvari Hrim Hrim Krim Krim Om*

# Strategic Naksatras for Dream Work

Two nakṣatras align particularly with dream practice.

Uttara Bhadrapada is ruled by Ahir Budhnya, the Serpent of the Depths. Its symbol-the back part of a funeral cot, or twin fish-represents the deep subconscious and the dream world.

Revati is ruled by Pusan the Nourisher. As the final naksatra, it governs transitions, including the passage from waking to the other side.

# The Twenty-Seven Beeja Mantras

*Table J.1. Naksatra beeja mantras.*

| Naksatra | Beeja Mantra | Naksatra | Beeja Mantra |
|---|---|---|---|
| Asvini | Om Am / Om Im | Svati | Om Am / Om Lam |
| Bharani | Om Im / Om Lim | Visakha | Om Yam / Om Ram |
| Krttika | Om Um / Om Vum | Anuradha | Om Num / Om Tham |
| Rohini | Om Rm / Om Lm | Jyestha | Om Dham / Om Nam |
| Mrgasira | Om Em / Om Vem | Mula | Om Am / Om Nam |
| Ardra | Om Aim / Om Tham | Purvasadha | Om Pam / Om Tham |
| Punarvasu | Om Om / Om Ham | Uttarasadha | Om Bham / Om Sam |
| Pusya | Om Aum / Om Sam | Sravana | Om Kham / Om Jham |
| Aslesa | Om Am / Om Gam | Dhanistha | Om Gam / Om Sam |
| Magha | Om Am / Om Ham | Satabhisaj | Om Sam / Om Am |
| Purva Phalguni | Om Im / Om Tham | Purva Bhadrapada | Om Sim / Om Dham |
| Uttara Phalguni | Om Um / Om Cham | Uttara Bhadrapada | Om Tham / Om Nam |
| Hasta | Om Rm / Om Jham | Revati | Om Am / Om Lam |
| Citra | Om Em / Om Ram | | |

# Application Methods

The Gatekeeper Method. Use the beeja mantra of the naksatra on the twelfth house cusp. The twelfth house represents exit from material world and entry into sleep; its naksatra lord acts as psychopomp for the dream state.

The Transit Method. Use the mantra for the current Moon naksatra. This aligns the subconscious with prevailing lunar weather.

The Pada Refinement. For specific internal alchemy or meridian-based dream work, use the syllable associated with the pada (the 3 degree 20 minute quarter) where the twelfth house cusp or natal

Moon sits. Example: if the cusp falls in the first pada of Asvini, the syllable is Chu.

Visualization. While chanting the beeja mentally, visualize the seed syllable glowing in soft moon-white light at the ajna cakra (third eye) to trigger transition into dreaming.

## Appendix K

# Mantras for Sleep and Dream Cultivation

*svapne suptasya ya devi sarvabhutesu samsthita | nidra-saktih samakhyata tasyai devyai namo namah*

*'That Goddess who abides in all beings as the power of sleep-to that Devi, salutations.'*

—Devi Mahatmyam 5.18

# I. Therapeutic Intention

The mantric protocols here address disturbances of the sleep-dream continuum through vibrational remediation. In Vedic understanding, sleep (*nidrā*) is not merely physiological rest but daily dissolution of individuated consciousness into its cosmic source-a rehearsal for the greater dissolution at death. Dream (*svapna*) occupies liminal territory between waking cognition and formless depths of deep sleep, serving as a theater where unprocessed impressions (samskaras) and karmic residues manifest as symbolic narrative.

When this natural rhythm is disturbed-whether through planetary affliction in the twelfth house, malefic aspects to the Moon, or constitutional imbalances affecting the manas (sensory mind)-Vedic tradition offers mantric intervention as primary therapeutic modality. These sound-formulas work through three mechanisms: they invoke protective deities (devata), they harmonize the vibrational signature of afflicting planets, and they anchor the wandering consciousness in sacred sound during the vulnerable transition into sleep.

# II. The Seven Rsis as Guardians of the Mind

The tradition of invoking Ṛṣis—the primordial seers who 'heard' the Vedas-for mental protection during sleep derives from their role as originators of specific Vedic hymns and their continued presence as stellar guardians. The seven principal Rsis correspond to the seven stars of Ursa Major (Saptarsi), understood in Jyotisa as the celestial council that governs cosmic order. Each Rsi presides over specific mental faculties and offers protection when that faculty is disturbed.

Invocation is performed before sleep, ideally after evening *sandhyā* (twilight worship) or, at minimum, after washing hands, feet, and face. The practitioner sits facing east or north, takes three conscious breaths, and recites the appropriate mantra 3, 9, or 27 times according to the severity of disturbance. The recitation should be neither rushed nor excessively prolonged; the traditional measure is one matra (unit) per syllable, roughly equivalent to the time required to snap one's fingers.

*Table K.1. Rsi invocations for sleep protection.*

| Rsi | Mantra | Indication | Governing Faculty |
|---|---|---|---|
| Atri | Om Atraye Namah | Lunar afflictions; emotional turbulence; vivid or disturbing dreams | Emotional mind (manas); Moon; Cancer |
| Vasistha | Om Vasistaya Namah | Self-doubt preventing sleep; performance anxiety; imposter syndrome | Self-confidence; Solar dignity; Leo |
| Kasyapa | Om Kasyapaya Namah | Fear of death; ancestral nightmares; past-life intrusions | Ancestral lineage; Saturn; eighth-house matters |
| Gautama | Om Gautamaya Namah | Intellectual overstimulation; racing thoughts; inability to turn off analytical mind | Discriminative intellect (buddhi); Mercury |
| Bharadvaja | Om Bharadvajaya Namah | Sleep disrupted by unfulfilled desires; restlessness from attachment | Desire and attachment; Venus; relationship axis |
| Visvamitra | Om Visvamitraya Namah | Anger-related insomnia; frustration; competitive drive preventing rest | Transformative will; Mars; Aries/Scorpio |
| Jamadagni | Om Jamadagnaye Namah | Spiritual seeking preventing rest; philosophical anxiety; crisis of meaning | Spiritual aspiration; Jupiter; Sagittarius/Pisces |

# III. Planetary Mantras for Twelfth-House Afflictions

When natal or transiting planets afflict the twelfth house or its lord, sleep disturbance follows a pattern characteristic of the afflicting *graha*. Saturn brings delayed sleep onset and early waking; Mars produces restless, aggressive dreams; Rahu generates anxiety and irrational fears at the sleep threshold; Ketu causes dissociative states and difficulty distinguishing dream from waking. The traditional remedy involves propitiating the afflicting planet through its specific mantric protocol.

Three classes of planetary mantras are employed in ascending potency. The bija (seed) mantras contain the compressed vibrational essence of the planet in a single syllable; they are potent but require precise pronunciation and should ideally be received from a qualified teacher. The pauranika (devotional) mantras invoke the planet as a deity, describing its attributes and seeking blessings; these are safer for general use. The Gayatri mantras petition for illumination and guidance from the planetary intelligence; they are particularly suited for transforming the quality of dream consciousness.

*Table K.2. Bija mantras for planetary afflictions.*

| Graha | Bija Mantra | Sleep-Related Indications |
|---|---|---|
| Surya (Sun) | Om Hram Hrim Hraum Sah Suryaya Namah | Lack of vitality upon waking; unrefreshing sleep; loss of circadian rhythm |
| Candra (Moon) | Om Sram Srim Sraum Sah Candraya Namah | Emotional dreams; lunar-cycle-related insomnia; maternal anxiety |
| Mangala (Mars) | Om Kram Krim Kraum Sah Bhaumaya Namah | Aggressive dreams; night sweats; teeth grinding; anger-disrupted sleep |
| Budha (Mercury) | Om Bram Brim Braum Sah Budhaya Namah | Racing thoughts; intellectual overstimulation; word-salad dreams |

| Graha | Bija Mantra | Sleep-Related Indications |
|---|---|---|
| Guru (Jupiter) | Om Gram Grim Graum Sah Gurave Namah | Prophetic dreams requiring interpretation; spiritual crisis; excessive sleep |
| Sukra (Venus) | Om Dram Drim Draum Sah Sukraya Namah | Sexual dreams; romantic longing; sleep disrupted by sensory indulgence |
| Sani (Saturn) | Om Pram Prim Praum Sah Sanaiscaraya Namah | Delayed sleep onset; early waking; nightmares of restriction; chronic fatigue |
| Rahu (North Node) | Om Bhram Bhrim Bhraum Sah Rahave Namah | Hypnagogic hallucinations; sleep paralysis; irrational nocturnal fears |
| Ketu (South Node) | Om Sram Srim Sraum Sah Ketave Namah | Dissociative states; confusion between dream and waking; karmic release dreams |

*Table K.3. Pauranika (devotional) mantras.*

The shorter devotional mantras are well-suited for bedside recitation. They require less precision than bija mantras while still invoking the planetary deity's presence. The recommended count is 108 repetitions using a mala (rosary), though 27 repetitions suffice when time is limited.

| Graha | Pauranika Mantra | Optimal Timing |
|---|---|---|
| Surya (Sun) | Om Ghrinih Suryaya Namah | Sunday; sunrise or before dawn |
| Candra (Moon) | Om Som Somaya Namah | Monday; moonrise or after sunset |
| Mangala (Mars) | Om Kum Kujaya Namah | Tuesday; morning hours |
| Budha (Mercury) | Om Bum Budhaya Namah | Wednesday; morning hours |
| Guru (Jupiter) | Om Brm Brhaspat aye Namah | Thursday; early morning (brahma muhurta) |
| Sukra (Venus) | Om Sum Sukraya Namah | Friday; evening hours |

| Graha | Pauranika Mantra | Optimal Timing |
|---|---|---|
| Sani (Saturn) | Om Sam Sanaye Namah | Saturday; after sunset |
| Rahu (North Node) | Om Ram Rahave Namah | Saturday; night hours |
| Ketu (South Node) | Om Kem Ketave Namah | Tuesday or Thursday; twilight |

*Table K.4. Gāyatrī Mantras for Dream Illumination.*

The gayatri meter carries a particular capacity for illuminating consciousness. Each planetary gayatri follows the structural template of the great Savitri (Rgveda 3.62.10), petitioning the deity to stimulate and guide the intellect. When employed for dream work, these mantras are recited during the transition into sleep with the intention that their illuminating quality persist into the dream state, fostering lucidity and meaningful revelation.

| Graha | Gayatri Mantra |
|---|---|
| Surya (Sun) | Om Bhaskaraya Vidmahe Divakaraya Dhimahi Tannah Suryah Pracodayat |
| Candra (Moon) | Om Ksiraputraya Vidmahe Amrtattvaya Dhimahi Tannah Candrah Pracodayat |
| Mangala (Mars) | Om Angarakaya Vidmahe Sakti dharaya Dhimahi Tanno Bhaumah Pracodayat |
| Budha (Mercury) | Om Gajadhvajaya Vidmahe Grahamadhyaya Dhimahi Tanno Budhah Pracodayat |
| Guru (Jupiter) | Om Vrsabhadhvajaya Vidmahe Grahasresthaya Dhimahi Tanno Guruh Pracodayat |
| Sukra (Venus) | Om Rajadabhaya Vidmahe Bhrgusutaya Dhimahi Tannah Sukrah Pracodayat |
| Sani (Saturn) | Om Kakadhvajaya Vidmahe Khadgahastaya Dhimahi Tannah Sanih Pracodayat |
| Rahu (North Node) | Om Nagadhvajaya Vidmahe Padmahastaya Dhimahi Tanno Rahuh Pracodayat |
| Ketu (South Node) | Om Asvadhvajaya Vidmahe Sulahastaya Dhimahi Tannah Ketuh Pracodayat |

# IV. Specific Mantras for Sleep Disorders

Beyond planetary framework, tradition preserves specific mantras addressed to deities presiding over sleep, dreams, and nocturnal protection. These may be employed independently or in combination with planetary protocols, particularly when the disturbance resists classification by graha influence alone.

*Table K.5. Devata Mantras for Sleep and Dream Protection.*

| Devata | Mantra | Application |
|---|---|---|
| Nidra Devi (Goddess of Sleep) | Om Hrim Nidradevyai Namah | General insomnia; difficulty entering sleep; resistance to rest |
| Ratri Devi (Goddess of Night) | Om Ratryai Namah | Fear of darkness; night anxiety; nocturnal panic |
| Visnu (Preserver) | Om Namo Narayanaya | Protection during sleep; nightmares; fear of attack |
| Hanuman (Protector) | Om Hanumate Namah | Nightmares; demonic dreams; spirit oppression; night terrors |
| Ganesa (Remover of obstacles) | Om Gam Ganapataye Namah | Sleep blocked by worry; mental obstacles to rest; pre-sleep anxiety |
| Durga (Fierce protectress) | Om Dum Durgayai Namah | Protection from malevolent influences; psychic attack; fear |
| Tara (Goddess who guides across) | Om Hrim Strim Hum Phat | Safe passage through dreams; lucid dreaming; nightmare transformation |
| Ksetrapala (Guardian of the field) | Om Ksam Ksetrapalaya Namah | Protection of sleeping space; warding; environmental disturbance |

# V. The Aditya Hrdayam for Anxiety-Related Insomnia

The *Āditya Hṛdayam* ('Heart of the Sun') holds unique position in the mantric pharmacopoeia for sleep disorders rooted in anxiety, depression, or loss of vital energy. This hymn appears in the Yuddha Kanda of the Ramayana, where the sage Agastya teaches it to Lord Rama on the battlefield, finding him exhausted and despairing before his confrontation with Ravana. The hymn restored Rama's courage, clarity, and vital force-a paradigm for its therapeutic application in states of mental and energetic depletion.

The complete hymn of 31 verses is traditionally recited at sunrise, though the condensed essence (verses 4-15) may be employed at any time for acute intervention. For sleep applications, evening recitation paradoxically promotes restful sleep by addressing the solar depletion underlying certain forms of insomnia-particularly the pattern of excessive fatigue coupled with inability to rest, common in states of burnout, grief, or chronic illness. The principle is one of restoration: by reconnecting with the solar source of vitality, the depleted individual can release into the lunar realm of sleep without the desperation that accompanies exhaustion.

The opening invocation may be employed as a standalone mantra:

*Om Hram Hrim Hraum Sah Aditya Hrdayaya Namah*

Therapeutic indication: insomnia arising from depletion, grief, loss of hope, seasonal affective patterns, or prolonged illness.

Contraindication: insomnia arising from excess heat, inflammation, or hyperactive states, where solar invocation may aggravate the condition.

# VI. Protocol Integration and Practical Application

Selection of appropriate mantras requires assessment through standard Jyotiṣa methodology: examination of the twelfth house, its lord, and occupants; the condition of the Moon and its dispositor; any malefic aspects or associations affecting these significators; and the current dasa-bhukti periods indicating activated karmic themes. The following decision tree provides a clinical framework:

*Step 1. Identify the primary afflicting planet through house occupancy, aspect, or rulership of the twelfth house or Moon. Address this planet with its bija or pauranika mantra.*

*Step 2. Assess the psychological quality of the disturbance and match to the appropriate Rsi invocation. Multiple Rsis may be invoked if the disturbance is compound.*

*Step 3. Consider supplementary devata mantras where specific protective or transformative qualities are indicated-Hanuman for nightmare patterns, Tara for lucid dreaming cultivation, etc.*

*Step 4. Observe the optimal timing indicated by planetary weekday and hour correspondences. While immediate need may override timing considerations, systematic practice aligned with muhurta principles deepens efficacy.*

*Step 5. Continue the selected protocol through the planetary period (mahadasa or antardasa) or for a minimum of 40 days to establish vibrational recalibration.*

Mantric approach integrates with, but does not replace, other therapeutic modalities. Sleep hygiene, herbal intervention, dietary adjustment, and-where indicated-professional medical consultation form the complete therapeutic context within which mantric practice operates.

# Sources

Coburn, Thomas B. *Devi-Mahatmya: The Crystallization of the Goddess Tradition*. Delhi: Motilal Banarsidass, 1984.

Frawley, David. *Mantra Yoga and Primal Sound: Secrets of Seed (Bija) Mantras*. Twin Lakes, WI: Lotus Press, 2010.

Harness, Dennis M. *The Nakshatras: The Lunar Mansions of Vedic Astrology*. Twin Lakes, WI: Lotus Press, 1999.

Kapoor, Gauri Shanker. *Remedial Measures in Astrology*. New Delhi: Ranjan Publications, 1995.

Rao, K. N. *Astrology, Destiny and the Wheel of Time*. New Delhi: Vani Publications, 1995.

*Ramayana of Valmiki*, trans. Robert P. Goldman et al., 7 vols. Princeton: Princeton University Press, 1984–2017.

Svoboda, Robert E. *The Greatness of Saturn: A Therapeutic Myth*. Twin Lakes, WI: Lotus Press, 1997.

Valmiki. *Aditya Hrdayam*, in *Yuddha Kanda* 105.1–31.

# Glossary

*Technical Terms in Oneiromancy, Astrology, and Traditional Medicine*

## Western Astrological Tradition

*Almuten (Arabic/Latin)*: From Arabic *al-mubtazz*, "the victor"; the planet with the greatest essential dignity at a specific degree, determined by summing points for domicile, exaltation, triplicity, term, and face.

*angular house*: Houses 1, 4, 7, and 10, positioned at the angles of the chart; planets in angular houses act with greatest strength and visibility.

*aspect*: A significant angular relationship between planets (conjunction 0°, sextile 60°, square 90°, trine 120°, opposition 180°); aspects to the 9th house ruler affect dream veracity.

*aversion*: Signs that cannot "see" each other—those in no Ptolemaic aspect relationship. Planets in aversion represent disconnected parts of the psyche requiring Gestalt dialogue to integrate.

*Bonatti, Guido*: Thirteenth-century Italian astrologer whose *Liber Astronomiae* codified medieval protocols for judging dream veracity through essential dignity assessment.

*cadent house*: Houses 3, 6, 9, and 12, positioned before the angles; the 9th house (cadent) governs long journeys, philosophy, religion, and dreams.

*cazimi (Arabic)*: A planet within 17′ of the Sun's center, considered to be "in the heart of the Sun" and greatly strengthened; contrasted with combustion.

*Chaldean order*: The traditional sequence of planets by apparent speed (Saturn, Jupiter, Mars, Sun, Venus, Mercury, Moon), used in calculating planetary hours and day rulerships.

*combust*: A planet within approximately 8° of the Sun, rendered invisible and weakened; a combust 9th house ruler diminishes dream reliability.

*detriment*: A planet positioned in the sign opposite its domicile; an essential debility reducing the planet's capacity to signify clearly.

*domicile*: A planet's "home" sign where it has greatest essential dignity (+5 points); e.g., Moon in Cancer, Saturn in Capricorn or Aquarius.

*Domus Dei (Latin)*: "House of God"; the traditional Latin designation for the 9th house, emphasizing its association with divine communication, prophecy, and dreams.

*Dorotheus of Sidon*: First-century CE astrologer whose *Carmen Astrologicum* preserved the Hellenistic triplicity lord system used in dream interpretation.

*electional astrology*: The branch of astrology concerned with selecting auspicious times for initiating activities; used to choose optimal moments for dream incubation.

*essential dignity*: A planet's intrinsic strength based on its zodiacal position; the five dignities are domicile (+5), exaltation (+4), triplicity (+3), term (+2), and face (+1).

*exaltation*: The sign where a planet is "exalted" or honored (+4 points); e.g., Sun in Aries (19°), Moon in Taurus (3°), Saturn in Libra (21°).

*face*: Also called decan; a 10° division of each sign, giving each planet rulership over specific faces (+1 point). The weakest essential dignity.

*fall*: A planet positioned in the sign opposite its exaltation; an essential debility indicating weakness or difficulty.

*firdaria (Persian)*: A planetary period system dividing life into segments ruled by different planets; used to identify which planetary themes dominate dream content during specific life phases.

*horary astrology*: The branch of astrology that answers specific questions by casting a chart for the moment the question is understood; dream charts are a form of horary practice.

*insomnium (Latin)*: In Macrobius classification, a nightmare or anxiety dream arising from physical or emotional disturbance; not prophetic but diagnostic of the dreamer's current state.

*Lilly, William*: Seventeenth-century English astrologer whose *Christian Astrology* (1647) systematized horary methods applicable to dream interpretation.

*Macrobius*: Fifth-century CE author whose Commentary on the Dream of Scipio established the fivefold classification of dreams (somnium, visio, oraculum, insomnium, visum) foundational to Western oneiromantic tradition.

*Lord of Divination*: The third (participating) triplicity lord of the 9th house, governing the native's intrinsic capacity for prophetic perception regardless of sect.

*Moon*: The primary significator of dreams in Western astrology; the Moon's condition, aspects, and void-of-course status are essential to dream judgment.

*oraculum (Latin)*: In Macrobius classification, a dream in which a respected figure (parent, priest, deity) delivers a direct message; the meaning is explicit.

*nativity (Latin)*: The birth chart; the horoscope cast for the moment of a person's birth, revealing constitutional tendencies including dream receptivity and prophetic capacity.

*participating lord*: The third triplicity ruler, governing the final third of life regardless of sect; when applied to the 9th house, becomes the Lord of Divination.

*profection (Latin)*: Annual house progression technique where the ascendant advances one sign per year of life; the profected house and its lord indicate dominant themes for that year, including dream content.

*peregrine*: A planet with no essential dignity at its current position; a peregrine 9th house ruler suggests dreams of uncertain origin or meaning.

*planetary hour*: A division of day and night into twelve unequal hours each, ruled by planets in Chaldean order; used for timing dream incubation, interpretation, and remedial work.

*reception*: The relationship between planets where one receives another into its dignity; reception between significators strengthens dream reliability.

*sect*: The distinction between diurnal (day) and nocturnal (night) charts based on the Sun's position relative to the horizon; affects triplicity lord assignments.

*significator*: A planet representing a specific person, topic, or question; the 9th house ruler is the primary significator for dreams.

*somnium (Latin)*: In Macrobius classification, an enigmatic prophetic dream requiring interpretation; the dream conceals its meaning in symbols that must be decoded.

*succedent house*: Houses 2, 5, 8, and 11, positioned after the angles; planets here act with moderate strength.

*term*: Also called bound; a division of each sign into five unequal segments ruled by different planets (+2 points). The Egyptian terms are most commonly used.

*visum (Latin)*: In Macrobius classification, a hypnagogic apparition occurring between waking and sleep; not prophetic.

*visio (Latin)*: In Macrobius classification, a prophetic dream that reveals future events literally as they will occur; no interpretation needed.

*tripartite night*: William Morris's application of triplicity structure to the nocturnal cycle: first third (processing daily experience), middle third (prophetic/psychic access), final third (preparation for waking).

*triplicity*: The grouping of signs by element (Fire, Earth, Air, Water); each triplicity has three planetary rulers (day, night, participating) governing different life periods.

*veracity*: The truthfulness or reliability of a dream's prophetic content; traditional astrology provides systematic criteria for assessment.

*void of course*: The Moon's condition when it makes no applying aspects before leaving its current sign; a void Moon at dream time may indicate a dream without significant outcome.

# Classical Chinese Medicine

*Dāntián 丹田*: Energy centers in internal alchemy; the Lower Dāntián (below the navel) is the focus of foundational cultivation practices and the settling point in sleep meditation.

*Dragon Bone (*Lóng Gǔ*)*: Fossilized bone used to anchor the spirit, astringe essence, and settle the Liver; key ingredient in formulas for spirit fragmentation and ghostly dreams.

*Fù Xíng Jué 輔行訣*: "Secrets for Auxiliary Cultivation"; manuscript attributed to Tao Hongjing preserving five-flavor organ therapeutics from the lost *Tāng Yè Jīng*.

*Gān Xuè Xū* 肝血虛: Liver Blood Deficiency; pattern causing unanchored *hún*, resulting in excessive dreaming, disturbed sleep, and difficulty remembering dreams.

*ghostly dream (*mèng yù guǐ jiāo*)*: Dreams of intercourse with ghosts; indicates fragmentation of self, leakage of essence, destabilization of spirit. Treated with Cinnamon Twig Decoction plus Dragon Bone and Oyster Shell.

*guǐ* 鬼: Ghost, demon, or disembodied spirit; contemporary euphemism for mental fixations, addictions, and erosion of psychological boundaries.

*Guī Pí Tāng* 歸脾湯: Restore the Spleen Decoction; formula for Spleen and Heart Blood deficiency with disturbed *shén*, indicated for anxiety, insomnia, and dream-disturbed sleep.

*Guì Zhī Jiā Lóng Gǔ Mǔ Lì Tāng*: Cinnamon Twig Decoction plus Dragon Bone and Oyster Shell; formula for spirit fragmentation, ghostly dreams, and boundary instability.

*Huángdì Nèijīng* 黃帝內經: The Yellow Emperor's Classic of Internal Medicine; foundational text containing earliest systematic discussion of dreams and the *wǔ shén*.

*hún* 魂: The ethereal soul, housed in the Liver and associated with Wood element and Jupiter. The *hún* travels during sleep, producing dreams; its proper anchoring in Liver Blood ensures peaceful dreaming. Primary generator of dream experience.

*jīng* 精: Essence; the most fundamental vital substance, stored in the Kidneys, governing constitution, reproduction, and the *zhì* spirit. Essence depletion produces fear dreams and dreams of loss.

*Língshū* 靈樞: The Spiritual Pivot; second section of the *Huángdì Nèijīng*, containing detailed discussion of the *wǔ shén* and diagnostic oneiromancy. Chapter 43 correlates dream content with organ pathology.

*Oyster Shell (*Mǔ Lì*)*: Used to subdue yang, soften hardness, and stabilize the Heart-Kidney axis; paired with Dragon Bone for anchoring the spirit.

*pò* 魄: The corporeal soul, housed in the Lungs and associated with Metal element and Venus. Enters with first breath, descends at death. Dreams involving strong physical sensation or instinct arise from the *pò*.

*pulse diagnosis*: Assessment of health through palpation of the radial artery; correlates dream content with pulse findings for integrated assessment.

*qì* 氣: Vital energy or life force; one of the vital substances whose circulation affects all organ functions including dream production.

*Sān Jiāo* 三焦: The Triple Burner; governs transformation and transportation of fluids and *qì* throughout the body.

*shén* 神: Spirit; specifically the spirit housed in the Heart and associated with Fire element and Mars. Governs consciousness, cognition, and integration of all psychic functions.

*Shèn Qì Wán*: Golden Cabinet Kidney Qi Pill; formula for Kidney Yang deficiency with difficulty exiting sleep.

*Sì Wù Tāng* 四物湯: Four Substances Decoction; base formula for Blood deficiency where unanchored *hún* produces disturbed dreaming.

*suān zǎo rén* 酸棗仁: Sour Jujube Seed (*Ziziphus jujuba* var. *spinosa*); nourishes Heart Blood and calms the *shén*, providing material basis for stable *hún* travel. Jupiter rulership.

*Sùwèn* 素問: The Basic Questions; first section of the *Huángdì Nèijīng*, establishing foundational theory including the relationship between Liver and *hún*.

*Tao Hongjing (456–536 CE)*: Liang dynasty scholar-hermit to whom the *Fù Xíng Jué* is attributed.

*Tāng Yè Jīng* 湯液經: Classic of Decoctions; lost text traditionally ascribed to Yi Yin, claimed source of the *Fù Xíng Jué* five-flavor therapeutics.

*Thirteen Ghost Points*: Acupuncture protocol developed by Sun Simiao (7th century) for spirit disturbance, possession states, mania, and deep-seated trauma.

*Tiān Wáng Bǔ Xīn Dān*: Emperor of Heaven's Special Pill to Tonify the Heart; formula for Yin deficiency with frequent waking.

*Tǐ-Yòng-Huà* 體用化: Substance-Function-Transformation; the *Fù Xíng Jué* paradigm differentiating whether organ pathology lies in substantial foundation, dynamic function, or capacity for transformation.

*Wēn Dǎn Tāng*: Warm the Gallbladder Decoction; formula for absent dream recall when phlegm mist obscures the dream landscape.

*wǔ shén* 五神: The Five Spirits: *hún* (Liver/Jupiter), *pò* (Lungs/Venus), *shén* (Heart/Mars), *yì* (Spleen/Saturn), *zhì* (Kidneys/Mercury). Each governs specific psychic functions and produces characteristic dream content when disturbed.

*wǔ wèi* 五味: The Five Flavors (sour, bitter, sweet, pungent/aromatic, salty); each performs different therapeutic functions depending on the element being treated.

*wǔ xíng* 五行: The Five Phases or Elements: Wood, Fire, Earth, Metal, Water. Each corresponds to specific organs, spirits, planets, and dream imagery.

*Xuè* 血: See Blood.

*yì* 意: The intellect or intention, housed in the Spleen and associated with Earth element and Saturn. Governs concentration, study, imagination. Spleen deficiency produces obsessive rumination and worry dreams.

*yīn/yáng* 陰/陽: The complementary polarities in Chinese cosmology. *Yīn* is associated with night, rest, and dream states; *yáng* with day, activity, and waking consciousness.

*Zhang Zhongjing*: Author of *Essentials from the Golden Cabinet* (c. 220 CE) containing the formula for ghostly dream treatment.

*zhì* 志: The will, housed in the Kidneys and associated with Water element and Mercury. Governs determination and drive to accomplish one's purpose. Kidney deficiency produces fear dreams, drowning dreams, paralysis of will.

## Daoist Internal Alchemy

*Organ Gaze*: Practice cultivating harmony among the five organ-spirits; warmth descends through the body, pausing at each organ in a generating cycle sequence.

*Liu Ming*: Contemporary Daoist teacher (Da Yuan Circle) who organized dream work into three layers: Healing, Divination, and Path. Developed the Night Meditation and Four Thresholds clinical approach.

*Neidān* 内丹: Internal alchemy; Daoist practices treating sleep as portal for ontological return rather than merely restoration.

*Shuì Gōng* 睡功: Sleeping Cultivation; Daoist practice treating sleep as the primary vehicle for spiritual cultivation and return to *Xiāntiān*.

*wúwéi* 無為: Non-action; the *Neidān* transition from *yǒuwéi* (doing) to *wúwéi* where mind and *qì* function naturally.

*Wújí* 無極: The Limitless; the Zero preceding the One in alchemical cosmogony, goal of ontological return through sleep practice.

*Xiāntiān* 先天: Pre-Celestial; the state before differentiation of Yin and Yang, goal of *Shuì Gōng* practice.

*yǒuwéi* 有為: Doing; the active phase of practice preceding the transition to *wúwéi*.

## Vedic Tradition (Jyotiṣa)

*Āruḍha Lagna*: The "image" of the ascendant, calculated by counting from the ascendant lord to its position and reflecting that distance; indicates the characteristic imagery, setting, and phenomenal quality of the dream experience.

*aśubha*: Inauspicious; imagery or timing that indicates unfavorable outcomes; contrasted with *śubha*.

*bhāgya*: Fortune, fate, or destiny resulting from merit or demerit in former existences; the ninth house governs *bhāgya*, linking dreams to karmic revelation.

*bhāva*: House in Vedic astrology; the twelve *bhāvas* correspond to different life domains, with the twelfth house governing dreams and sleep.

*Broken Dream Principle*: Teaching that if a dreamer wakes and returns to sleep, the dream loses prophetic charge; the circuit is broken and the message fails to ground.

*Construction Chart*: Technique for analyzing complex dreams by manually placing planets in houses based on dream narrative content, creating a symbolic horoscope capturing the dream's internal logic.

*dāna*: Charitable giving; a remedial measure for planetary affliction. Mercury *dāna* includes educational donations and green cloth.

*daśā*: A planetary period system assigning rulership over specific life phases; the *Viṃśottari daśā* (120-year cycle) is most commonly used. Dream charts employ a compressed version scaled to twelve months.

*Deva nakṣatra*: Lunar mansions of divine temperament, producing benevolent dream content, spiritual guidance, and good omens.

*gaṇa*: Temperament classification of *nakṣatras*: *Deva* (divine), *Manuṣya* (human), or *Rākṣasa* (demonic); indicates the quality of dreams occurring under each lunar mansion.

*guna (Sanskrit)*: Quality or attribute; the three gunas (sattva, rajas, tamas) govern mental states and affect dream clarity. Sattva predominates in the fourth watch, producing the clearest prophetic dreams.

*graha*: Planet; literally "seizer," reflecting the understanding that planets grasp or influence terrestrial affairs.

*Harṣa Yoga*: Joy Combination; twelfth lord in the twelfth house, the ideal configuration for sound sleep.

*janma nakṣatra*: The lunar mansion occupied by the natal Moon; when the Moon at dream time matches this mansion, significance deepens.

*Jyotiṣa*: Vedic astrology, the "science of light"; locates dream signification primarily in the 12th house and uses *nakṣatras* for timing interpretation.

*kāraka*: Significator; a planet naturally signifying a particular domain. Jupiter is *kāraka* for dreams; Ketu is *Mokṣa Kāraka* (Significator of Liberation).

*karma*: The accumulated consequences of past actions across lifetimes; karmic patterns manifest through dreams, particularly those involving the 12th house.

*karma nakṣatra*: The tenth mansion from natal Moon; addresses vocation and life purpose when the Moon transits this position at dream time.

*Ketu*: The South Node of the Moon; associated with past-life patterns, spiritual liberation, latent pathogens, and epidemic influence. Ketu in the twelfth thins the veil between worlds; natives report astral travel, lucid dreaming, encounters with deceased.

*kīṭa*: Insect, worm, or parasite; associated with Ketu, indicating infection or parasitic patterns that may manifest through dream imagery.

*lagna*: The Ascendant; the sign rising on the eastern horizon. Represents the essential self and point of incarnation.

*mahāpuruṣa yoga*: Great Planetary Combination; when a planet occupies its own sign or exaltation in an angular house, creating strength that may manifest through characteristic dream content.

*Manuṣya nakṣatra*: Lunar mansions of human temperament, producing dreams of ordinary concerns, work, family, worldly matters.

*maraṇa kāraka sthāna*: A position of "death-like weakness" for a planet; affects the reliability of that planet as a dream significator.

*Mokṣa Trikoṇa*: Liberation Triangle; houses 4, 8, and 12, governing the soul's journey beyond material existence.

*nakṣatra*: One of 27 lunar mansions, each spanning 13°20′ of the zodiac; provide detailed timing and symbolic content for dream interpretation. Three temperamental groups: *Deva, Manuṣya, Rākṣasa.*

*Navāṃśa*: The Ninth Divisional Chart; Sun-Moon connections for dream validation may appear here if not in the *Rāśī* chart.

*niṣphala*: Futile; a dream rendered non-predictive by interruption or disturbed conditions (illness, intoxication, exhaustion).

*Praśna Mārga*: Classical text on horary astrology; establishes that when crucial events approach, the ninth lord activates dream communication.

*preta*: Hungry ghost; entity in an intermediate state between death and rebirth. *Preta-doṣa* (ancestral ghost affliction) manifests through dreams of incomplete communication with the deceased.

*Rāhu*: The North Node of the Moon; associated with worldly desire, obsession, foreignness, and amplification. Rāhu in the twelfth intensifies dreams to the point of confusion; sleep paralysis and night terrors correlate with Rāhu's presence.

*Rākṣasa nakṣatra*: Lunar mansions of demonic temperament, producing difficult imagery, conflict, ancestral demands, karmic weight.

*rāśi*: Sign of the zodiac; measured sidereally rather than tropically.

*śrāddha*: Ancestral ceremony; ritual offerings to deceased relatives performed to honor ancestors and resolve *preta-doṣa* indicated through dreams.

*śubha*: Auspicious; imagery or timing that indicates favorable outcomes; contrasted with *aśubha*.

*Sūrya*: The Sun; solar dreams feature blazing fire, royalty, temples, gold, governmental authority.

*svapna*: The dream state and its contents; recognizes that mode of consciousness and its productions cannot be separated.

*upāya*: Remedial measure prescribed to address planetary afflictions; may include mantras, gemstones, charity, or ritual actions indicated by dream analysis.

*Varāhamihira*: Sixth-century CE polymath whose *Bṛhat Saṃhitā* devotes several chapters to dream interpretation within its encyclopedic treatment of omen science.

*Viṃśottari daśā*: The most commonly used planetary period system, based on a 120-year cycle. Dream charts employ compressed version scaled to twelve months.

*Vyaya Bhāva*: House of Loss; the twelfth house, governing sleep, dreams, and what must be surrendered for sleep to occur.

*yāma*: A night watch; the division of the night into four three-hour periods (*prahara*), each with distinct predictive ranges. First watch (sunset–10 PM): manifestation within one year. Fourth watch (3 AM–sunrise): manifestation within ten days to immediate.

## Greco-Roman Tradition

*allegorical dream*: In Artemidorus's classification, a dream requiring symbolic interpretation, where the manifest content differs from the latent meaning; contrasted with theorematic dreams.

*Artemidorus of Daldis*: Second-century CE author of the *Oneirocritica*; established the foundational classification of dreams into *enhypnion* and *oneiros*, and further divided prophetic dreams into theorematic and allegorical types.

*Asclepius*: Greek god of medicine whose temples (*Asclepieia*) served as centers for therapeutic dream incubation; son of Apollo, trained by Chiron.

*abaton (Greek)*: The innermost sacred chamber of an Asclepian temple where supplicants slept to receive healing dreams; from Greek ἄβατον, "not to be entered" (by the uninitiated).

*enkoimesis (Greek)*: The practice of ritual sleep in a sacred precinct to receive divine dreams; from Greek ἐγκοίμησις, "sleeping in."

*enhypnion (Greek)*: A non-prophetic dream arising from present physical or emotional states; mental housekeeping. Contrasted with *oneiros*.

*kline (Greek)*: The sacred couch or sleeping platform in an Asclepian *abaton* where supplicants received healing dreams.

*oneirocritica (Greek)*: The science or art of dream interpretation; title of Artemidorus's systematic treatise.

*oneiros (Greek)*: A prophetic dream pointing to future events; stirs the soul and demands interpretation. Contrasted with *enhypnion*.

*theorematic dream*: A dream whose meaning is identical to its manifest content; literal fulfillment. Contrasted with allegorical dreams.

## Mesopotamian Tradition

*asû (Akkadian)*: Therapeutic physician; practitioner focused on physical symptoms through herbal and surgical treatments.

*bārû (Akkadian)*: Seer; diviner who read omens and interpreted dreams.

*Gula (Akkadian)*: Goddess patroness of medicine; bridged the realms of physical treatment and spiritual healing.

*Iškar Zaqīqu (Akkadian)*: The Assyrian Dream Book; eleven tablets preserving dream interpretation employing linguistic puns revealing the deep structure of reality.

*Namburbi (Akkadian): Apotropaic ritual to avert consequences of unfavorable omens,* including bad dreams; the dream reveals tendency, not inevitable outcome.

*šā›ilu (Akkadian)*: Questioner; dream diviner who might be an *āšipu*, *bārû*, or ecstatic prophet.

*šammu ša šamê šubatšu (Akkadian)*: "The plant whose home is heaven"; formula recognizing oneirogens as operating on both physical and spiritual registers.

*Uruanna (Akkadian)*: Pharmacological lexicon containing approximately 1,300 terms describing some 340 plants used in medical and ritual practice.

*zaqīqu (Akkadian)*: Dream-Spirit; entity who delivers messages during incubation.

## Egyptian Tradition

*Duat*: The Netherworld through which Ra journeys nightly; the sleeping soul participates in this descent and rebirth.

*Nun*: The Primordial Waters from which creation emerged; vast dark water in dreams indicates contact with the source—fertile potential and formless chaos at once.

*Ra*: Sun god who sails across the sky by day and descends to fight Apophis in the Duat by night, reborn at dawn. Dreams participate in this nocturnal journey.

## Islamic Tradition

*ta'wīl (Arabic)*: The science of dream interpretation; seeking hidden meaning beneath manifest content.

## Tibetan Buddhist Tradition

*Milam: Dream yoga practices train the practitioner to recognize the dream state, transform dream content, and recognize the luminous nature of the* mind.

*lungta (Tibetan)*: Wind horse; the vital force governing forward momentum, confidence, and auspicious movement. Dreams of flying or swift travel indicate strong lungta; dreams of being stuck indicate depletion.

*mewa (Tibetan)*: The nine magic square numbers cycling through years, months, and days; each carries specific qualities and bardo implications affecting dream practice and interpretation.

*parkha (Tibetan)*: The eight trigrams adapted from Chinese ba gua; govern directions, spatial orientation, and sleeping positions for dream yoga practice.

*rigpa (Tibetan)*: Pure awareness; the luminous nature of mind equally present in waking, dreaming, and deep sleep. Recognition of rigpa is the ultimate aim of dream yoga practice.

*srog (Tibetan)*: Life force; the vital energy sustaining existence. When srog is weak, dreams turn toward death, dissolution, and endings.

## Aboriginal Australian Traditions

*Tjukurrpa (Western Desert languages)*: The "Dreamtime" or "Dreaming"; the eternal, ever-present reality in which ancestor spirits created the land and continue to inhabit it. Not past but ongoing.

## African Traditions

*n|om (Ju|'hoan)*: Among the Kalahari San, the spiritual energy or "medicine" activated through trance dance; boiling *n|om* enables visionary experience.

*sangoma (Zulu/Xhosa)*: Traditional healer or diviner whose calling (*ubizo*) often comes through dreams; uses *ubulawu* preparations for ancestral communication.

*Silene capensis (Latin)*: African Dream Root (*undlela ziimhlophe*, "white paths"); primary oneirogen of southern African *ubulawu* tradition. Saturn rulership. Used for ancestral communication.

*ubulawu (Zulu/Xhosa)*: Dream-inducing plant medicines used in traditional diviner initiation; prepared as foaming decoctions.

*undlela ziimhlophe (Xhosa)*: "White paths"; name for African Dream Root describing the roads along which ancestors travel.

# Hawaiian Tradition

*moe 'uhane*: Soul Sleep; the soul (*'uhane*) leaves the body during sleep to travel and receive messages from *'aumakua*.

*'uhane*: Soul; leaves the body during *moe 'uhane* to travel and receive ancestral messages.

*'aumakua (Hawaiian)*: Ancestral guardian spirits; family deities who communicate through dreams during moe 'uhane (soul sleep), offering guidance, warnings, and protection.

# Mesoamerican Tradition

*thle-pelakano (Chontal Maya)*: "Leaf of god"; the Chontal Maya name for Calea zacatechichi (Dream Herb), used for divinatory dreaming and receiving prophetic visions. See Calea zacatechichi under General Terms.

# Western Alchemical Tradition

*albedo (Latin)*: The whitening stage following nigredo; Moon's stage. Dreams of purification, washing, dawn light, silver, and lunar imagery indicate this phase.

*citrinitas (Latin)*: The "yellowing" stage; represents solar consciousness awakening, the emergence of gold. Sun's stage.

*coniunctio (Latin)*: The "sacred marriage" of opposites (masculine/feminine, conscious/unconscious); represents psychological integration.

*nigredo (Latin)*: The "blackening" stage; Saturn's stage. Dreams of death, decay, descent, dismemberment. The old self dies. These dreams feel like failure, but signal that transformation has begun.

*Rubedo (Latin)*: The "reddening" stage; represents integration, the union of red king and white queen, phoenix rising. The Self manifests.

## Depth Psychology

*Empty Chair*: Classic Gestalt technique placing an empty chair before the dreamer, who alternately occupies their own position and that of dream figures, conducting dialogue to integrate projected aspects.

*felt sense*: In Focusing, bodily awareness of meaning that precedes conceptual articulation; the body's knowing is used to verify dream interpretations.

*Focusing*: Technique developed by Eugene Gendlin using the body's knowing as a guide to interpretation; involves six movements: clearing a space, felt sense, handle, resonating, asking, receiving.

*Gendlin, Eugene (1926–2017)*: Philosopher and psychotherapist who developed Focusing from research into why some therapy clients improved while others did not.

*Gestalt method: Dream interpretation technique developed by Fritz Perls in which the dreamer speaks as each dream element in the* first person present tense, treating all images as projected aspects of the psyche.

*Lucid dreaming*: The state of being aware that one is dreaming while the dream continues; techniques for inducing lucidity have cross-cultural precedents.

*object catalog*: Technique systematically inventorying all dream elements (objects, figures, animals, colors, actions, settings, sensations) before proceeding to interpretation; prevents overlooking quieter details.

*Perls, Fritz*: Developer of Gestalt therapy and the Empty Chair technique for dream work.

# Oneirobotany (Materia Medica)

*Celastrus paniculatus (Latin)*: Intellect Tree (*jyotiṣmatī*); Āyurvedic *medhya rasāyana* that ensures the dreamer returns with the message intact—Mercury rulership.

*Laurus nobilis (Latin)*: Bay Laurel; sacred to Apollo, ruled by Sun. Provides prophetic clarity; where Mugwort opens gates, Bay illuminates what is encountered.

*Mandragora officinarum (Latin)*: Mandrake; Akkadian *nam-tar* ("fate-cutter"). Saturn rulership (root), Venus (fruit). Contains tropane alkaloids, producing profound sedation. TOXIC.

*medhya rasāyana (Sanskrit)*: Intellect-Rejuvenating Substances in Āyurveda; enhance cognitive function, including dream recall and clarity.

*Mugwort (*Artemisia vulgaris*)*: The preeminent oneirogen of the Northern Hemisphere. Moon rulership. Thujone acts as a GABA receptor antagonist, maintaining cortical awareness during REM.

*Nymphaea caerulea (Latin)*: Blue Lotus; sacred in Egyptian iconography. Venus rulership. Contains apomorphine and nuciferine, which affect dopamine receptors.

*oneirogen*: Dream-inducing; substances that facilitate access to the dream realm without overwhelming waking consciousness. From Greek *óneiros* (dream) and *-gen* (producing).

*Polygala tenuifolia (Latin)*: *Yuǎn zhì* ("far-reaching will"); opens Heart orifices blocked by phlegm—Mercury rulership.

*Withania somnifera (Latin)*: Ashwagandha; species name means "sleep-bearing." Adaptogen normalizes stress response and supports natural sleep architecture. Saturn/Mars rulership.

*Ziziphus jujuba var. **spinosa** (Latin)*: See *suān zǎo rén* under Classical Chinese Medicine.

## General Terms

*incubation*: The deliberate practice of seeking significant dreams through ritual preparation, prayer, and sleeping in sacred locations; from Latin *incubare*, "to lie upon."

*apotropaic*: Rituals or objects intended to avert evil or misfortune; from Greek ἀποτρόπαιος, "turning away." In Mesopotamian dream practice, apotropaic rituals nullified unfavorable dream portents.

*Bardo Thödol (Tibetan)*: "Liberation Through Hearing in the Intermediate State"; the Tibetan Book of the Dead. Describes consciousness navigating the bardo states between death and rebirth; lucid dreaming practice prepares for this transition.

*Calea zacatechichi (Latin)*: Dream Herb; Chontal Maya oneirogen used for divinatory dreaming. Called *thle-pelakano*, "leaf of god." Jupiter/Mercury rulership.

*chthonic (Greek)*: About the underworld or earth depths; from χθών, "earth." Chthonic dreams involve descent, ancestral contact, or encounters with underworldly figures.

*extispicy*: Divination by examining animal entrails, especially the liver; from Latin *exta*, "entrails." Mesopotamian divinatory practice was parallel to oneiromancy; the *bārû* (seer) often practiced both arts.

*hypnagogic*: The transitional state between wakefulness and sleep; from Greek ὕπνος, "sleep," and ἀγωγός, "leading." Hypnagogic imagery often carries symbolic significance. Compare *hypnopompic*, the transition from sleep to waking.

*Jukurrpa (Warlpiri)*: The Dreaming; Aboriginal Australian cosmological concept of the eternal creative epoch accessible through dreams and ceremony. Also, *Tjukurrpa* in Western Desert languages.

*MILD*: Mnemonic Induction of Lucid Dreams, a technique developed by Stephen LaBerge involving pre-sleep intention-setting and affirmation to achieve dream lucidity.

*numinous*: Having a quality of sacred mystery or divine presence; from Latin *numen*, "divine will." Rudolf Otto developed the term; numinous dreams carry archetypal weight and transformative potential.

*paranomasia (Greek)*: Wordplay or punning used as an interpretive technique; from παρονομασία, «play on words.» The core method in Mesopotamian dream interpretation, preserved in the Iškar Zaqīqu, linguistic puns revealed the deep structure of reality.

*WILD*: Wake Initiated Lucid Dream; technique maintaining conscious awareness through the hypnagogic transition directly into the dream state without loss of lucidity.

*oneiromancy*: Divination through the interpretation of dreams; from Greek ὄνειρος (*oneiros*, "dream") and μαντεία (*manteia*, "prophecy").

*prophetic dream*: A dream conveying accurate information about future events; traditional systems provide criteria for assessing prophetic reliability.

# Bibliography

## Primary Sources: Western Astrological Texts


Abū Ma'shar al-Balkhī. *The Abbreviation of the Introduction to Astrology*. Edited and translated by Charles Burnett. Leiden: Brill, 1994.

Abū Ma'shar al-Balkhī. *The Great Introduction to Astrology*. Translated by Keiji Yamamoto and Charles Burnett. 2 vols. Leiden: Brill, 2019.

al-Bīrūnī, Abū Rayḥān. *The Book of Instruction in the Elements of the Art of Astrology*. Translated by R. Ramsay Wright. London: Luzac, 1934.

Bonatti, Guido. *Liber Astronomiae*. Translated by Benjamin N. Dykes. 3 vols. Minneapolis: Cazimi Press, 2007.

Dorotheus of Sidon. *Carmen Astrologicum*. Translated by David Pingree. Leipzig: Teubner, 1976.

Firmicus Maternus. *Mathesis*. Translated by Jean Rhys Bram. Park Ridge, NJ: Noyes Press, 1975.

Lilly, William. *Christian Astrology*. London, 1647. Reprint, Exeter: Regulus, 1985.

Manilius. *Astronomica*. Translated by G. P. Goold. Loeb Classical Library. Cambridge, MA: Harvard University Press, 1977.

Māshā'allāh. *On Reception*. Translated by Benjamin N. Dykes. Minneapolis: Cazimi Press, 2010.

Ptolemy. *Tetrabiblos*. Translated by F. E. Robbins. Loeb Classical Library. Cambridge, MA: Harvard University Press, 1940.

Sahl ibn Bishr. *The Introduction to the Science of the Judgments of the Stars*. Translated by Benjamin N. Dykes. Minneapolis: Cazimi Press, 2008.

Vettius Valens. *Anthologies*. Translated by Mark Riley. Self-published, 2010.

## Primary Sources: Vedic and Sanskrit Texts

*Bṛhat Jātaka of Varāhamihira*. Translated by N. Chidambaram Iyer. Madras: South Indian Press, 1885.

*Bṛhat Saṃhitā of Varāhamihira*. Translated by M. Ramakrishna Bhat. Delhi: Motilal Banarsidass, 1981.

Jaimini. *Jaimini Sūtras*. Translated by P. S. Sastri. New Delhi: Ranjan Publications, 1992.

Parāśara. *Bṛhat Parāśara Horā Śāstra*. Translated by R. Santhanam. 2 vols. New Delhi: Ranjan Publications, 1984.

*Praśna Mārga*. Translated by B. V. Raman. Bangalore: IBH Prakashana, 1991.

*Swapna Adhyāya* [Dreams chapter]. In *Bṛhat Saṃhitā*. Translated by M. Ramakrishna Bhat. Delhi: Motilal Banarsidass, 1981.

## Primary Sources: Ancient Dream Texts

Artemidorus. *Oneirocritica*. Translated by Robert J. White. Park Ridge, NJ: Noyes Press, 1975.

Ibn Sīrīn. *Ta'bīr al-Ru'yā* [The Interpretation of Dreams]. Various Arabic editions.

Macrobius. *Commentary on the Dream of Scipio*. Translated by William Harris Stahl. New York: Columbia University Press, 1952.

Oberhelman, Steven M., ed. *Dreambooks in Byzantium: Six Oneirocritica in Translation, with Commentary and Introduction*. Aldershot: Ashgate, 2008.

Oppenheim, A. Leo. "The Interpretation of Dreams in the Ancient Near East." *Transactions of the American Philosophical Society* n.s. 46, no. 3 (1956): 179–373.

Zhou Gong. *Zhou Gong Jie Meng* [Duke of Zhou's Dream Interpretations]. Traditional Chinese text, various editions.

## Primary Sources: Chinese Medical Texts

*Huangdi Neijing Lingshu. Ling Shu, or The Spiritual Pivot.* Translated by Wu Jing-Nuan. Washington, DC: Taoist Center, 1993.

*Huangdi Neijing Suwen. Huang Di Nei Jing Su Wen: Nature, Knowledge, Imagery in an Ancient Chinese Medical Text.* Translated by Paul U. Unschuld and Hermann Tessenow. Berkeley: University of California Press, 2011.

*Huangdi Neijing Suwen. The Yellow Emperor's Classic of Internal Medicine—Simple Questions.* Translated by Ni Maoshing. Boston: Shambhala, 1995.

Li Shi-Zhen. *Bin Hu Mai Xue* [The Lakeside Master's Study of the Pulse]. Various translations.

*Nanjing. Nan-Ching: The Classic of Difficult Issues.* Translated by Paul U. Unschuld. Berkeley: University of California Press, 1986.

Sun Si-Miao. *Bei Ji Qian Jin Yao Fang* [Essential Prescriptions Worth a Thousand Gold]. Tang Dynasty, 652 CE.

*Yì Zōng Jīn Jiàn* [Golden Mirror of Medical Orthodoxy]. *Tang Ye Jing* [Classic of Decoctions] sections. Qing Dynasty compilation, 1742.

## Secondary Sources: Astrological Scholarship

Barton, Tamsyn. *Ancient Astrology.* London: Routledge, 1994.

Brennan, Chris. *Hellenistic Astrology: The Study of Fate and Fortune.* Denver: Amor Fati Publications, 2017.

DeFouw, Hart, and Robert Svoboda. *Light on Life: An Introduction to the Astrology of India.* London: Arkana, 1996.

Dykes, Benjamin N. *Traditional Astrology for Today: An Introduction.* Minneapolis: Cazimi Press, 2011.

Hand, Robert. *Night and Day: Planetary Sect in Astrology.* Orleans, MA: ARHAT Publications, 1995.

Pingree, David. *From Astral Omens to Astrology: From Babylon to Bīkāner.* Rome: Istituto Italiano per l'Africa e l'Oriente, 1997.

Rath, Sanjay. *Jyotiṣa Fundamentals*. New Delhi: Sagar Publications, 2014.

Rath, Sanjay. "Interpretation of Dreams: Jyotiṣa Methods." Lecture series, Śrī Jagannātha Centre, 2018–2022.

Rochberg, Francesca. *The Heavenly Writing: Divination, Horoscopy, and Astronomy in Mesopotamian Culture*. Cambridge: Cambridge University Press, 2004.

Zoller, Robert. *The Arabic Parts in Astrology: A Lost Key to Prediction*. Rochester, VT: Inner Traditions, 1989.

## Classical and Ancient Studies

Edelstein, Emma J., and Ludwig Edelstein. *Asclepius: Collection and Interpretation of the Testimonies*. 2 vols. Baltimore: Johns Hopkins University Press, 1945. Reprint, 1998.

Graf, Fritz. *Magic in the Ancient World*. Translated by Franklin Philip. Cambridge, MA: Harvard University Press, 1997.

Butler, Sally A. L. *Mesopotamian Conceptions of Dreams and Dream Rituals*. Münster: Ugarit-Verlag, 1998.

Harris, W. V. *Dreams and Experience in Classical Antiquity*. Cambridge, MA: Harvard University Press, 2009.

Meier, Carl Alfred. *Healing Dream and Ritual: Ancient Incubation and Modern Psychotherapy*. Einsiedeln, Switzerland: Daimon Verlag, 1989.

Maul, Stefan M. "How the Babylonians Protected Themselves against Calamities Announced by Omens." In *Mesopotamian Magic: Textual, Historical, and Interpretive Perspectives*, edited by Tzvi Abusch and Karel van der Toorn, 123–29. Groningen: Styx, 1999.

Miller, Patricia Cox. *Dreams in Late Antiquity: Studies in the Imagination of a Culture*. Princeton, NJ: Princeton University Press, 1994.

Price, Simon. "The Future of Dreams: From Freud to Artemidorus." *Past and Present* 113 (1986): 3–37.

Scurlock, JoAnn, and Burton R. Andersen. *Diagnoses in Assyrian and Babylonian Medicine*. Urbana: University of Illinois Press, 2005.

## Secondary Sources: Chinese Medicine

Bensky, Dan, Steven Clavey, and Erich Stöger. *Chinese Herbal Medicine: Materia Medica*. 3rd ed. Seattle: Eastland Press, 2004.

Deadman, Peter, Mazin Al-Khafaji, and Kevin Baker. *A Manual of Acupuncture*. Hove, UK: Journal of Chinese Medicine Publications, 2007.

Flaws, Bob. *The Secret of Chinese Pulse Diagnosis*. 2nd ed. Boulder, CO: Blue Poppy Press, 1995.

Hammer, Leon. *Chinese Pulse Diagnosis: A Contemporary Approach*. Rev. ed. Seattle: Eastland Press, 2005.

Jarrett, Lonny S. *Nourishing Destiny: The Inner Tradition of Chinese Medicine*. Stockbridge, MA: Spirit Path Press, 1998.

Maciocia, Giovanni. *The Foundations of Chinese Medicine: A Comprehensive Text for Acupuncturists and Herbalists*. 2nd ed. Edinburgh: Churchill Livingstone, 2005.

Maciocia, Giovanni. *The Psyche in Chinese Medicine: Treatment of Emotional and Mental Disharmonies with Acupuncture and Chinese Herbs*. Edinburgh: Churchill Livingstone, 2009.

Morris, William. *Neoclassical Pulse Diagnosis*. Self-published, 2020.

Morris, William. *Li Shi-Zhen Pulse Studies*. Self-published, 2021.

Rossi, Elisa. *Shen: Psycho-Emotional Aspects of Chinese Medicine*. Edinburgh: Churchill Livingstone, 2007.

Unschuld, Paul U. *Medicine in China: A History of Ideas*. Berkeley: University of California Press, 1985.

Wiseman, Nigel, and Feng Ye. *A Practical Dictionary of Chinese Medicine*. 2nd ed. Brookline, MA: Paradigm Publications, 1998.

## Depth Psychology

Freud, Sigmund. *The Interpretation of Dreams*. Translated by James Strachey. New York: Basic Books, 1955.

Gendlin, Eugene. *Focusing*. New York: Everest House, 1978.

Jung, C. G. *Dreams*. From *The Collected Works of C. G. Jung*, vols. 4, 8, 12, and 16. Translated by R. F. C. Hull. Princeton, NJ: Princeton University Press, 1974.

Jung, C. G. *Man and His Symbols*. New York: Doubleday, 1964.

Jung, C. G. *Memories, Dreams, Reflections*. Recorded and edited by Aniela Jaffé. Translated by Richard and Clara Winston. New York: Vintage Books, 1963.

LaBerge, Stephen. *Lucid Dreaming: The Power of Being Awake and Aware in Your Dreams*. Los Angeles: Jeremy P. Tarcher, 1985.

Perls, Frederick. *Gestalt Therapy Verbatim*. Lafayette, CA: Real People Press, 1969.

Moss, Robert. *Conscious Dreaming: A Spiritual Path for Everyday Life*. New York: Crown, 1996.

Stevens, Anthony. *Private Myths: Dreams and Dreaming*. Cambridge, MA: Harvard University Press, 1995.

Van de Castle, Robert L. *Our Dreaming Mind*. New York: Ballantine Books, 1994.

Wangyal Rinpoche, Tenzin. *The Tibetan Yogas of Dream and Sleep*. Ithaca: Snow Lion, 1998.

## Cross-Cultural Dream Studies

Bulkeley, Kelly. *Dreaming in the World's Religions: A Comparative History*. New York: New York University Press, 2008.

Cumes, David. *Africa in My Bones: A Surgeon's Odyssey into the Spirit World of African Healing*. Cape Town: New Africa Books, 2004.

Eliade, Mircea. *Shamanism: Archaic Techniques of Ecstasy*. Translated by Willard R. Trask. Princeton, NJ: Princeton University Press, 1964.

Fabricius, Johannes. *Alchemy: The Medieval Alchemists and Their Royal Art*. Copenhagen: Rosenkilde and Bagger, 1976.

Halifax, Joan. *Shamanic Voices: A Survey of Visionary Narratives*. New York: Dutton, 1979.

Irwin, Lee. *The Dream Seekers: Native American Visionary Traditions of the Great Plains*. Norman: University of Oklahoma Press, 1994.

Katz, Richard. *Boiling Energy: Community Healing among the Kalahari Kung*. Cambridge, MA: Harvard University Press, 1982.

Keeney, Bradford, and Hillary Keeney. *Way of the Bushman: Spiritual Teachings and Practices of the Kalahari Ju|'hoansi*. Rochester, VT: Bear & Company, 2015.

Moss, Robert. *Dreamways of the Iroquois: Honoring the Secret Wishes of the Soul*. Rochester: Destiny Books, 2005.

Ngubane, Harriet. *Body and Mind in Zulu Medicine*. London: Academic Press, 1977.

O'Flaherty, Wendy Doniger. *Dreams, Illusion, and Other Realities*. Chicago: University of Chicago Press, 1984.

Pukui, Mary Kawena, E. W. Haertig, and Catherine A. Lee. *Nānā I Ke Kumu*. 2 vols. Honolulu: Hui Hānai, 1972.

Shulman, David, and Guy G. Stroumsa, eds. *Dream Cultures: Explorations in the Comparative History of Dreaming*. New York: Oxford University Press, 1999.

Stanner, W. E. H. *The Dreaming and Other Essays*. Melbourne: Black Inc. Agenda, 2009.

Somé, Malidoma Patrice. *Of Water and the Spirit*. New York: Penguin, 1994.

Szpakowska, Kasia. *Behind Closed Eyes: Dreams and Nightmares in Ancient Egypt*. Swansea: Classical Press of Wales, 2003.

Tedlock, Barbara, ed. *Dreaming: Anthropological and Psychological Interpretations*. Cambridge: Cambridge University Press, 1987.

Young, Serinity. *Dreaming in the Lotus: Buddhist Dream Narrative, Imagery, and Practice*. Boston: Wisdom Publications, 1999.

## Nakṣatras and Vedic Astrology

Bepin Behari. *Myths and Symbols of Vedic Astrology*. Salt Lake City: Passage Press, 1990.

Frawley, David. *Astrology of the Seers: A Guide to Vedic/Hindu Astrology*. Twin Lakes, WI: Lotus Press, 2000.

Harness, Dennis M. *The Nakshatras: The Lunar Mansions of Vedic Astrology*. Twin Lakes, WI: Lotus Press, 1999.

Kane, Pandurang Vaman. *History of Dharmaśāstra*. Vol. 4. Poona: Bhandarkar Oriental Research Institute, 1953.

Rath, Sanjay. *Collected Papers in Vedic Astrology*. Vol. 1, chapter 12, "Interpretation of Dreams." New Delhi: Sagar Publications, 2007.

Sutton, Komilla. *The Nakshatras: The Stars Beyond the Zodiac*. Bournemouth, UK: Wessex Astrologer, 2014.

Wilhelm, Ernst. *Graha Sutras*. Kala Occult Publishers, 2006.

## Philosophy of Mind and Soul

Bremmer, Jan N. *The Early Greek Concept of the Soul*. Princeton, NJ: Princeton University Press, 1983.

Copenhaver, Brian P. *Hermetica: The Greek Corpus Hermeticum and the Latin Asclepius in a New English Translation*. Cambridge: Cambridge University Press, 1992.

Dodds, E. R. *The Greeks and the Irrational*. Berkeley: University of California Press, 1951.

Shaw, Gregory. *Theurgy and the Soul: The Neoplatonism of Iamblichus*. University Park: Pennsylvania State University Press, 1995.

## Ethnobotany and Materia Medica

Grieve, Maud. *A Modern Herbal*. 2 vols. New York: Dover Publications, 1971. Originally published 1931.

Emboden, William A. "The Sacred Narcotic Lily of the Nile." *Economic Botany* 32 (1978): 395–407.

Frawley, David, and Vasant Lad. *The Yoga of Herbs*. Twin Lakes: Lotus Press, 2001.

Hirst, Manton. "Dreams and Medicines: Xhosa Diviners." *Indo-Pacific Journal of Phenomenology* 5 (2005): 1–22.

Mayagoitia, Lidia, et al. "Psychopharmacologic Analysis of *Calea zacatechichi*." *Journal of Ethnopharmacology* 18 (1986): 229–243.

Rätsch, Christian. *The Encyclopedia of Psychoactive Plants: Ethnopharmacology and Its Applications*. Translated by John R. Baker. Rochester, VT: Park Street Press, 2005.

Sobiecki, Jean-François. "Psychoactive Ubulawu Spiritual Medicines and Healing Dynamics in the Initiation Process of Southern Bantu Diviners." *Journal of Psychoactive Drugs* 44, no. 3 (2012): 216–223.

Wood, Matthew. *The Earthwise Herbal: A Complete Guide to Old World Medicinal Plants*. Berkeley: North Atlantic Books, 2008.

Wood, Matthew. *The Earthwise Herbal: A Complete Guide to New World Medicinal Plants*. Berkeley: North Atlantic Books, 2009.

## Scriptural and Religious Sources

Genesis 28:12–17; 37:5–11; 40:1–23; 41:1–36. New Revised Standard Version.

Homer. *Iliad*. Translated by Richmond Lattimore. Chicago: University of Chicago Press, 1951.

Homer. *Odyssey*. Translated by Richmond Lattimore. New York: Harper & Row, 1967.

Plato. *Republic*. Translated by G. M. A. Grube, revised by C. D. C. Reeve. Indianapolis: Hackett, 1992.

Plato. *Timaeus*. In *Complete Works*, edited by John M. Cooper. Indianapolis: Hackett, 1997.

# About the Author

William Morris, DAOM, PhD, is a scholar-practitioner with a clinical career spanning forty-five years. Since beginning his practice in 1980, he has focused on the transdisciplinary synthesis of the celestial arts and East Asian medicine, a framework he defines as "Sky Medicine."

*The Book of Dreams* is Volume IX in the Sky Medicine series, a comprehensive integration of medical astrology, Classical Chinese Medicine, and traditional healing arts. Other volumes address pulse diagnosis, herbal therapeutics, life-arc assessment, and the confluence of meridian and celestial systems.

At the heart of his approach is a sophisticated weaving of Hellenistic, Vedic, and Chinese astrological techniques. By integrating these diverse systems, Dr. Morris develops assessment models that align the "Music of the Spheres" with the somatic realities of the clinic. This method utilizes planetary cycles, fixed stars, and the subtle elements to inform herbal strategies and provide a deeper understanding of the patient's psycho-emotional and spiritual landscape.

In this volume, he bridges these astrological traditions with Daoist internal alchemy *(Neidan)*, specifically drawing upon the sleep and dream practices of Chen Tuan and Zhang Jingyue. Through this lens, the astrological chart becomes a map of the spirit, and the clinical encounter becomes an act of harmonizing the dreamer with celestial patterns that shape both illness and awakening.

Made in the USA
Monee, IL
11 September 2026

60956657R00217